COUNSELING
MEN

THE BROOKS/COLE SERIES IN COUNSELING PSYCHOLOGY
John M. Whiteley, University of California at Irvine
Arthur Resnikoff, University of California at Irvine
Series Editors

Helene K. Hollingsworth
Editorial Assistant

APPROACHES TO ASSERTION TRAINING
Editors: John M. Whiteley, University of California at Irvine
        John V. Flowers, University of California at Irvine
THE BEHAVIOR THERAPIST
Editor: Carl E. Thoresen, Stanford University
CAREER COUNSELING
Editors: John M. Whiteley, University of California at Irvine
        Arthur Resnikoff, University of California at Irvine
COUNSELING ADULTS
Editors: Nancy K. Schlossberg, University of Maryland
        Alan D. Entine, State University of New York at Stony Brook
COUNSELING MEN
Editors: Thomas M. Skovholt, University of Minnesota
        Paul G. Schauble, University of Florida at Gainesville
        Richard Davis, The Western Ohio Council for Educational and
            Behavioral Programs – Lima, Ohio
COUNSELING WOMEN
Editors: Lenore W. Harmon, University of Wisconsin-Milwaukee
        Janice M. Birk, University of Maryland
        Laurine E. Fitzgerald, University of Wisconsin-Oshkosh
        Mary Faith Tanney, University of Maryland
DEVELOPMENTAL COUNSELING AND TEACHING
Editors: V. Lois Erickson, University of Minnesota
        John M. Whiteley, University of California at Irvine
THE HISTORY OF COUNSELING PSYCHOLOGY
Editor: John M. Whiteley, University of California at Irvine
THE PRESENT AND FUTURE OF COUNSELING PSYCHOLOGY
Editors: John M. Whiteley, University of California at Irvine
        Bruce R. Fretz, University of Maryland
THEORETICAL AND EMPIRICAL FOUNDATIONS OF
    RATIONAL-EMOTIVE THERAPY
Editors: Albert Ellis, Institute for Rational-Emotive Therapy
        John M. Whiteley, University of California at Irvine

COUNSELING MEN

EDITED BY

THOMAS M. SKOVHOLT
UNIVERSITY OF MINNESOTA

PAUL G. SCHAUBLE
UNIVERSITY OF FLORIDA

RICHARD DAVIS
THE WESTERN OHIO COUNCIL FOR
EDUCATIONAL AND BEHAVIORAL PROGRAMS,
LIMA, OHIO

BROOKS/COLE PUBLISHING COMPANY
MONTEREY, CALIFORNIA

A DIVISION OF WADSWORTH, INC.

Dedicated to
Cathy, Betty, and Carol

Acquisition Editor: *Claire Verduin*
Project Development Editor: *Ray Kingman*
Production Editor: *Stacey C. Sawyer*
Interior Design: *Laurie Cook*
Cover Design: *Sharon Marie Bird*
Typesetter: *Lehmann Graphics*

Printed in the United States of America

10 9 8 7 6 5 4 3 2 1

Much of the material in this book originally appeared in *The Counseling Psychologist*, the official publication of the Division of Counseling Psychology of the American Psychological Association.

Library of Congress Cataloging in Publishing Data
Main entry under title:

Counseling men.

   (Brooks/Cole series in counseling psychology)
   Bibliography:
   Includes index.
   1. Men—Counseling.   2. Sex role.   3. Men—Mental
health.   I. Skovholt, Thomas M.   II. Schauble, Paul G.
III. Davis, Richard, 1945–
RC451.4.M45C68   362.8   79-29722
ISBN 0-8185-0372-6

SERIES FOREWORD

The books in the Brooks/Cole Series in Counseling Psychology reflect the significant developments that have occurred in the counseling field over the past several decades. No longer is it possible for a single author to cover the complexity and scope of counseling as it is practiced today. Our approach has been to incorporate within the Brooks/Cole Series the viewpoints of different authors having quite diverse training and perspectives.

Over the past decades, too, the counseling field has expanded its theoretical basis, the problems of human living to which it addresses itself, the methods it uses to advance scientifically, and the range of persons who practice it successfully—from competent and skillful paraprofessionals to doctoral-level practitioners in counseling, psychology, education, social work, and psychiatry.

The books in the Brooks/Cole Series are intended for instructors and both graduate and undergraduate students alike who want the most stimulating in current thinking. Each volume may be used independently as a text to focus in detail on an individual topic, or the books may be used in combination to highlight the growth and breadth of the profession. However they are used, the books explore the many new skills that are available to counselors as they struggle to help people learn to change their behavior and gain self-understanding. Single volumes also lend themselves as background reading for workshops or in-service training, as well as in regular semester or quarter classes.

The intent of all the books in the Brooks/Cole Series is to stimulate the reader's thinking about the field, about the assumptions made regarding the basic nature of people, about the normal course of human development and the progressive growth tasks that everyone faces, about how behavior is acquired, and about what different approaches to counseling postulate concerning how human beings can help one another.

John M. Whiteley
Arthur Resnikoff

PREFACE

An intensive interest in sex roles has developed during the last several years. Researchers and theorists in this area hope that the examination of sex roles will provide a rich, new perspective in the behavioral sciences. Much of the recent research and theorizing, however, has focused on the behavior of females. The articles in this volume represent the less well-developed literature that focuses on the behavior of males. The authors have examined the facets of the male experience—as through a prism—in order to illuminate information, concepts, and strategies useful to counselors and psychotherapists.

In the first essay, Art Hansen and Tom Skovholt look at the big picture of male socialization and behavior by examining major trends in the current shifting of sex roles. They offer a new perspective on sex-role changes and discuss troublespots for males.

The next article is a piece by Joe Pleck, a leader in the study of male behavior. Pleck offers some intriguing ideas on a central male/female issue: power.

Jack Crites and Louise Fitzgerald use T.A. language in the ensuing article to create a new perspective on male psychological competence.

The next two articles examine male sexual behavior. Alan Gross explains patterns in male heterosexual behavior; Joseph Norton focuses on homosexuality as an alternative style of male sexuality.

Bob Lewis follows with an article on emotional intimacy among men. He suggests that male role behavior limits closeness between men, and he argues for changes in male behavior.

Jerry Toomer examines males in psychotherapy both as clients and as therapists. He reviews a number of studies on the effect of the sex variable on process and outcome research, and he asks a number of important therapy-related questions.

Monty Bruch joins Toomer in addressing the question practitioners often ask while kibitzing in the office: why don't men come for counseling as often as women do? Bruch also examines John Holland's theory on career development, and he spins a number of related sophisticated research questions and intervention ideas.

Bob Chapman discusses young males. He asks why boys experience three to four times more emotional difficulties than young girls and suggests causes and solutions.

James Savage and Yvonne Kelley shed light on the concerns of Black males and show that ethnicity influences male behavior in general.

The next two articles explore two topics that exist because of male involvement: rape and impotence. Therapists Mike Stockton, Denise Edwards, and Brainard Hines consider sexual offenses, not from the usual perspective—that of the victim—but from the viewpoint of offenders, and they suggest some overall strategies for counseling men. Barry McCarthy writes about secondary impotence, a problem that some observers say is increasing as sex roles change.

The last six articles examine male roles in the family. As an increasing number of women move away from homemaking as their central adult task, many people are showing interest in family roles for men. Mike Berger and Larry Wright feature this topic: they question whether breadwinning is the only compatible family role for men, and they suggest public changes to encourage male involvement in the family.

Jean Gearing extends the discussion of family roles to include childbirth, an event that usually has more significance for women, and she campaigns for extending the bonding between parent and child to include father/child as well as mother/child bonding. Jaquie Resnick, Mike Resnick, Athol Parker, and Jen Wilson expand on Gearing's theme by discussing fathering. They suggest systematic parent-education programs for men.

The next two articles are devoted to the effect on fathers of the loss of their children. Bob Woody looks at the difficult but important problem of custody of children after divorce. John Wanzenreid considers the equally important topic of caring for men after a major loss—the death of a child. He uses a case of Sudden Infant Death to explore the subject of male grief.

In the final article, David Rice draws on his clinical experience to offer a number of ideas for practitioners to consider when working with male clients in marriage and family therapy.

During the editing of this book we realized that the choice of some topics invariably excluded other equally important areas for exploration. However, we feel that the following essays will provide useful additions to the literature in professional psychology and will be especially useful in advanced courses in counseling. Specifically, we hope that the counseling and psychotherapy services provided to boys and men will be enhanced by the content of this volume.

Thomas M. Skovholt
Paul G. Schauble
Richard Davis

CONTENTS

INTRODUCTORY ARTICLE 1

Men's Development: A Perspective and Some Themes

THOMAS M. SKOVHOLT
University of Minnesota

ART HANSEN
University of Florida

The traditional rules and expectations concerning men's and women's behavior are changing dramatically in our society and many others. Statuses and roles, economic values, salary and wage scales, legal and religious codes and practices, character traits, career goals, and personal styles and desires—all of these, insofar as they express supposed differences between men and women, are being examined and re-evaluated.

A high level of affect is being generated by this current reappraisal of sex-related rules and behavior. Every type of emotion seems to be aroused: hope and despair, fear and tranquility, anger and joy, resentment and appreciation. Most of all, the burning of old blueprints for our lives brings anxiety, the kind of anxiety experienced by the traveler who goes on a crucial journey with a map that is known to be outdated.

The order of authorship of this article was determined randomly.

This article addresses three questions: What are the major changes in men's lives? What is causing and sustaining these changes? How are men reacting to the changes in their and in women's lives?

The majority of visible changes involve women and their roles. Women are moving into areas that were previously reserved for men, and women are changing the rules that regulate their behavior. These changes range from economic to symbolic, sexual to religious, play to deadly earnest.

Women are working as carpenters, repairmen (repair persons?), bankers, politicians, clergy, and astronauts. They are demanding equal pay and promotion. Other areas of change are primarily important as expressions of symbolic inequality and restriction that influence personal motivation and pride; three areas include codes of dress and etiquette, beauty contests and linguistic terms of reference and address (examples of these terms are Ms., his/her, chair/chairman/chairperson of a meeting, and assumption of a husband's last name on marriage).

Young women are engaging in vigorous athletic events and are competing as members of mixed-sex teams. In athletics and sexuality women are playing more and more by what used to be men's rules. In more deadly areas women are becoming police officers, soldiers and sailors in the armed services, are attending military academies and are being assigned to hazardous duties.

Women are seen as the direct instigators of these changes, and their motivation is easily understandable. The fields they are moving into are valued and rewarded, and women have been prevented from participation of the basis of their sex. Character traits and personal styles that have been associated with career success and personal freedom have been associated traditionally with men. In order to succeed in male-dominated work arenas, women are adopting traditional male patterns and simultaneously denying the male-only association of those patterns.

ACCOMMODATIVE CHANGES IN MEN'S LIVES

Men's lives are also changing, although with less public attention and drama. One of the reasons why these changes are less apparent is that they are not primarily concerned with new economic activities for men. Some movement into women's traditional work and workplaces has occurred, it is true, as men have become house husbands, male nurses, or kindergarten teachers. But the emphasis for most men is in learning how to live in different ways with the women in their lives, both in workplaces where only men used to be and in the more intimate areas of sexuality and marriage.

The primary changes in men's lives are accommodative. The changes are reactions and adjustments to innovations in women's behavior and expectations. These accommodations to women-initiated innovations include changes in men's styles and attitudes, in the quality of sexual relationships, and in the allocation of tasks at work and at home. These changes are important but less publicly obvious than changes in role assignment. For most men in our society work and the workplace are central in their adult lives. Most of the energies and ambitions of men are focused on work and career. Much of their time is spent working away from home, and many of their associations are with people met at work, although the contacts may continue outside the workplace in bars, parties, and recreation. Whether a farm, an office, or a factory, the places, the companions, and the conversation are generally male oriented. Women are generally in supporting roles as secretaries or assistants and are spatially separated and in lower-paid positions.

As women are moving up in rank and responsibility, however, the workplace is becoming integrated.There is no longer an all-male cast. Traditional male styles (including the humor) are less appropriate in this new environment, and men at work are devising and experimenting with new ways to act and interact.

Homes are women's domains. Men fit into them as enforcers and consumers—disciplining the children and eating the meals. There are specifically male tasks and niches: taking care of the car and taking out the garbage, being responsible for electricity and mechanics, occupying dens and workshops and easy chairs, doing the heavy lifting, and enjoying a reputed lordship, but the essential daily home duties are women's. They purchase and process food and clothing, clean and arrange the house and oversee the children. One reason retirement for men is traumatic is because they exchange significant activity in male-dominated places for inactivity in places dominated by their wives.

Accommodative changes in men's lives are also occurring at home and as fathers. Wives and women friends who work outside the home are unable and often unwilling to continue assuming full responsibility for food, clothing, and other household tasks and major responsibility for raising the children.

Two options are available. One involves negotiating new divisions of labor in which men and children assume the responsibility for various household jobs. The other option involves reducing absolutely the amount of household labor handled by the family. Processed foods are purchased or the family eats out more. Who cooks at your home: mom, dad, or Ronald McDonald? People to clean the house are hired part-time, and clothes are sent to laundries. Many couples combine aspects of both options.

These domestic changes alter the content of men's lives and boys' socialization. What is the sense of home for men? A castle, a haven to retire to after the day's work, a place to be waited on by a woman—these idealistic images do not accurately reflect the real home life of more traditional families, but the images portray ideals that are goals and models men hold in their minds. Changes in the images and expectations of work-place and home are difficult to measure but culturally and psychologically critical.

Boys are the next generation of men. The world these boys grow up in is normal for them. It is in this way that innovations for one generation become traditions for the next. The changes in socialization are easily exaggerated, however, since the major changes are restricted to women's economic activities. Many sexually attributed character traits and behavior patterns that are not economically related are being traditionally transmitted to today's children. It is the authors' impression that the division in preferences between clothes and dolls for girls and athletics and guns for boys still continues less changed than children's ideas and expectations about future career possibilities.

REASONS FOR MEN TO SUPPORT CHANGE

We have stressed the term *accommodative* because most of the changes mentioned above are in response to women-initiated actions. Because of the importance and chronological priority of feminist pressure, a common assumption is that men's traditional lives would not change if women stopped their sometimes-organized, sometimes-spontaneous campaigns. We disagree with this simplistic understanding of the forces impelling change.

It is undoubtedly true that women are the major direct impetus for change. If women stopped demanding, the rate of change would diminish (and, in some specific areas, stop immediately). This reflects the fact that the changes in sexual behavior and ideas have not been an equal convergence of men and women toward androgyny or any other synthesis. Instead the changes have been much more lopsided with women adopting more nontraditional (for women) behaviors and attitudes than men.

Although this is true, the movement has progressed enough by this time that there is a significant male input. Feminists and others have advanced the study of sex and gender beyond the attack on male privilege to explore the ways in which both men and women are restricted and traumatized by the rules, conflicts, and contradictions of our traditional ways of living.

The exploration of male anxieties and troublespots provides ample evidence that there are reasons for men to support the movement away from traditional male roles and character development. The existence of these problems and snakepits is becoming common knowledge. More men are now conscious of these negative aspects of becoming and being manly.

As men address their own lives, seeking a different self-realization than the traditional one, they also contribute to the pressure for change. By now enough men are doing this that, without any additional feminine pressure, these men will continue on their own to change themselves and offer alternative models for male development.

It is appropriate to review here some of these major problem areas for men. We are not stating that men have a higher rate of emotional difficulties than women. Whether there are sex differences in such rates is currently an issue in the journals. Common wisdom suggests that women suffer more often; the data are unclear. It seems to depend on whether antisocial, aggressive behaviors are considered part of emotional difficulties (Dohrenwend & Dohrenwend, 1976, 1977; Gove & Tudor, 1973, 1977).

1. The Elementary School Years

If we look at two groups, group A and group B, and realize that group A as a whole thrives and group B as a whole fails to thrive, then we begin to ask: What is wrong with the experience of Group B? In elementary school, girls are in group A and boys in group B (Tooley, 1977). Study after study after study reveals that boys experience approximately 75% of the difficulty and turmoil while girls experience only 25% (Eme, 1979; Grambs & Waetjen, 1975, p. 123; Werry & Quay, 1971).

The early years are difficult years for many boys. Most boys survive their early negative experiences and become competent adults; for others the negative experiences produce major effects throughout their lives.[1] What explains this great differential between the negative experiences of young boys and young girls? The answer seems to involve a complex nature/nuture interaction in which the variance is impossible to parcel out.

Child psychiatrist Richard Miner (Note 1) cautions against a strong nurture explanation. He suggests that the sex chromosomal disadvantage of males results in males being more vulnerable throughout the life cycle. Of sixty-four specific causes of death, males exceed females in all but seven (Lerner, 1968, p. 120). Many more male than female embryos are aborted or stillborn. At four months of embryonic age there are approximately 300 male embryos to each 100 female embryos; at birth there are 106 males to each 100 females; at age sixty-seven there are 70 males to each 100 females; at age one hundred there are 21 males to each 100 females (Lerner, 1968, p. 120). These biological facts may help explain difficulties young boys experience with death rates ⅓ higher than girls (Lerner, 1968, p. 120), with short attention spans and distractability (Werry & Quay, 1971), as well as with hyperactivity, dyslexia, and learning problems (Levy, Note 2).

---

[1]Some have suggested that the maternal-type rejection boys experience is, in the long run, positive. Boys learn independence behavior through defiance, but girls usually do not. Consequently, years later, many adult females are struggling with issues of defiance, independence, and assertion long after boys have learned how to reject authority figures and survive emotionally.

A second explanation is more environmental. Little boys are socialized first by women (mothers and teachers) but, in contrast to little girls, little boys must break away from women as a same-sex model and find men to model. There are few to be found! Father often has the career accelerator pushed to the floor and is not around, and the people at school are predominantly female. Schools seem to be female territory. In one study second-grade students said neutral objects (blackboards, books, school desks) were feminine (Kagan, 1964).

Difficulties with the demands for conformity and passivity seem to result from the multiplication of two factors. Boys have a higher level of physical energy and activity. Boys also have stronger demands for sex-appropriate behavior than girls.The differential in demands is often summarized by the example that girls are permitted to be tomboys while boys are not permitted to be sissies. In addition, since few adult males are around for boys to model, they tend to rely on male peers who often enforce rigorous, stereotypic male behavior. The result is a strongly physically aggressive style that schools often punish, sometimes by labelling it as an indication of an intellectual or emotional problem.

In school boys are punished for *not being* boys and also are punished for *being* boys. Grambs and Waetjen (1975) write:

> Teachers give boys more attention than girls in elementary school classrooms—but the attention is punitive. . . . The bias against boys in grading has been documented for over sixty years. . . . It is small consolation to know that it is men who . . . hold the destiny of the world in their hands if you just happen to be one of the millions of boys whom the system has defeated. . . . Is there another country in which society expects one kind of sex-appropriate behavior and the state-controlled educational system demands and rewards the antithesis? . . . After receiving poor grades, a boy may be prevented from having access to advanced work. Boys receive assaults on their self-concept by being labeled slow, stupid or dull. . . . It is astounding that parents and teachers permit such social and personal injustice. Is it that we expect men to have touble in life, to become defiant, to suffer failure, that we educate them to make these things more likely to happen [pp. 125–127]?[2]

As a solution Grambs and Waetjen (1975, p. 168) suggest that simply infusing elementary schools with more men teachers is naive. The bigger arena is the clash of expectations for boys between the larger society (be belligerent and tough and active) and the school (be quiet and obedient and still). They say either sex role expectations or school expectations must change.

Still it is somewhat of a puzzle why the affirmative action programs to increase the number of women professors in higher education in order to promote the development of women students has not taken a foothold in a reverse way at the elementary level. Perhaps the comparative lack of money and status is the answer, or perhaps the elimination of sex role stereotyping has not reached this issue because it is not a feminist issue.

2. *The Fallout from Adolescent Male Aggressiveness*

The aggressive male style that is an element of school problems is itself a continuing problem area. We both *applaud* and *condemn* the physical aggressiveness of male children, teenagers, and adults. Men the hunters, men the killers, men the strong, men the fierce—these aggressive roles and character traits are sometimes encouraged and other times discouraged.

Among all known human societies men have been the pool from which warriors were recruited. For us seventeen is the perfect age for conscription. It is the age when young men are physically mature and psychologically eager to display their courage and toughness, to prove themselves as men. We select these men to fight our countless battles and go up the countless hills: from San Juan Hill to Hamburger Hill and beyond. The carnage of young men in this century alone runs into the tens of thousands. Why these men do it is a question seldom asked even in the sex role literature.

Most of the answer is obviously cultural and social. Strength in men is positively valued. War and violence are institutionalized as means and mechanism for self-defense and -aggrandizement. Life is perceived as a struggle; resources are limited; there is an ethic of Social Darwinism.

Athletics and other forms of competition are also expressions of this positive evaluation. In this country football is the ongoing metaphor for combat. Millions attend games or tune in their television sets to sportsmanship and the knocking of heads on the gridiron. Although Robinson Jeffers' philosophy is an unusual one, his poem "The Bloody Sire" is particularly appropriate to cite here as a statement of value.

It is not bad. Let them play.
Let the guns bark and the bombing-plane
Speak his prodigious blasphemies.
It is not bad, it is high time,
Stark violence is still the sire of all the world's values.

What but the wolf's tooth whittled so fine
The fleet limbs of the antelope?
What but fear winged the birds, and hunger
Jeweled with such eyes the great goshawk's head?
Violence has been the sire of all the world's values.

Who would remember Helen's face
Lacking the terrible halo of spears?
Who formed Christ but Herod and Caesar,
The cruel and bloody victories of Caesar?
Violence, the bloody sire of all the world's values.

Never weep, let them play,
Old violence is not too old to beget new values.[3]

Another part of the answer lies in social organization. Older men have the resources to punish and reward the younger. The old men direct; the young fight and die. War is a game that old men play with younger men as pawns and pieces. We, the authors, believe that negotiation rather than combat would be employed to solve territorial disputes if military conscription started at fifty years of age instead of seventeen.

Death in war or sport is not the only trap of violence for men. Another trap of violence also awaits those socialized as warriors. Societies are extremely cautious about violence . The key is to know and practice only appropriate (as socially defined) forms. A year ago one of the authors taught in a Florida prison. There he was astonished to find a number of inmates who were Vietnam veterans.

This trap is open for all young men. Just as readily as we applaud their aggression we also strongly condemn it. The sly fox, the big wolf, and the blue jay are symbols here. For young men the line is thin between applause and condemnation. It is easy for a young man to commit enough antisocial acts in one day to be sent away for a long time: get high, rob a store with a rifle, steal a car, take a hostage, have a high speed chase, and then prison for 5 . . . 10 . . . 15 years. And it happens all the time. Eighty-three percent of the people arrested in 1970 were male (Noblet & Burcart, 1976).

The line is thin for many young men, but the line is thicker for a few others. Those that trespass greatly are remembered: David Berkowitz, Arthur Bremmer, Gary Gilmore, Charles Manson, Sirhan Sirhan, Richard Speck, and Charles Starkweather.

Prisons in Florida house 14 men for each woman. Some say that rehabilitation in the prisons is essentially one of time. Forty-year-old males do not commit the impulsive aggressive acts of younger men and, except for repeated offenders who are part of a criminal subculture, most men after 35 are simply less physically aggressive. Arnold Mandell in *Coming of Middle Age* (1977) suggests a brain chemistry explanation.

The last violent trap we will mention is accidental. Homicide is now the leading cause of death for 24- to 34-year-old nonwhite males. Accidents are second (Rushforth, Ford, Hirsch, Rushforth, & Adelson, 1977). When young females drink and drive they usually drive slower. When young

[3]"The Bloody Sire," by Robinson Jeffers. Copyright 1940 and renewed 1968 by Donnan Jeffers and Garth Jeffers. Reprinted from *The Selected Poetry of Robinson Jeffers*, by permission of Alfred A. Knopf, Inc.

males drink and drive they usually drive faster. So the fatalities caused by young male drivers of cars or motorcycles is high. In one study, 99% of the motorcycle fatalities were males. Their median age was 25: half were legally intoxicated (Baker & Fisher, 1977).

3. Restrictive Emotionality

Although we have presented two other problem areas before this one, restrictive emotionality is the most often cited male troublespot in the literature. The titles of books and articles point to it: Fasteau (1974) and *The Male Machine;* Goldberg (1977) and *The Hazards of Being Male;* Jourard (1974) and "Some lethal aspects of the male role"; and Balswick and Peek (1976) and "The inexpressive male: A tragedy of American society." David and Brannon (1976) subtitle two sections of their book "The sturdy oak: A manly air of toughness, confidence, and self-reliance" and "Give 'em hell: The aura of aggression, violence, and daring." Bem (1975b), exploring androgyny, uses the expression chesty. Alan Alda (1975), the actor, call it testosterone poisoning.

Traits traditionally considered positive for men include toughness, rationality, objectivity, dominance, aggression, self-reliance, and anger, while negatively valued ones include tenderness, emotional sensitivity, indecision, passivity, compassion, dependence, openness to experience, and vulnerability.

The idea of an ecological balance can be applied to understanding male emotionality. Some varieties of emotional expression are appropriate for the traditional male role, while others are not. If the male role requires competitive and violent behavior as in hand-to-hand combat, then qualities of the heart such as empathy would be immobilizing because empathy tends to reduce aggression (Deardorff, Finch, Kendall, Lira, & Indrisano, 1975). For example, empathy training is used in treating sex offenders (Stockton, Edwards, & Hines, 1979).

Male socialization demands that boys learn what are appropriate sentiments. Adults of both sexes and the boy's peers share in punishing "sissy-type" behaviors while rewarding manliness. "Socialization practices in respect to the boy have emphasized that the expression of grief over pain is babyish and unmanly. Further, experiencing pain and inflicting it on others is presented as 'fun' for the boy . . . " (Tooley, 1977, p. 189). A male client told one of the authors that the message he got from his best male friends in high school was "show any weakness and we'll kill you." The adult world for men continues the enforcement. "Corporate work stimulates and rewards qualities of the head and not the heart" (Maccoby, 1976, p. 176).

Traditional male socialization thus produces men who often find it difficult to easily develop emotional friendships with other men. A variety of factors seem to interrelate.

Men uniformly self-disclose less than women (Jourard, 1971). This restriction makes it difficult for men to get to know each other and become friends. Most often, it is only in unusual moments of great joy or sorrow that men are self-disclosing. Examples include a usually tough belligerent coach, Al McGuire, weeping openly as his Marquette University basketball team won the NCAA championship in 1977. A second incident occurred recently when one of the authors came upon a car accident in which a young baby was cut and bleeding from the head. Both mother and father were identically distraught and immobilized by the injury to their baby. Such emotionality is unusual for men.

Male competitiveness is another factor. Males often see the world as made up of winners and losers. If they win someone loses, and if they lose someone wins. Tooley (1977) summarizes:

> No wonder the civilized virtues of compromise, conciliation and open-ness to the ideas, needs and desires of others are, in practice, so often and so easily discarded; male psychology perceives these qualities as feminine 'submissiveness' and 'passivity'—as emasculation. Fear of emasculation, whether expressed as the boyhood fear of castration or the grownup male fear of impotence, remains the core organizer of adult male life experience [p. 191].

Many men live by a two-pronged belief: (1) relationships with other men are essentially competitive, and (2) one does not become vulnerable or reveal oneself to competitors.

Yet another factor is homophobia. The sexual discomfort that an intense male/male friendship sometimes generates functions to keep many men from easily developing these friendships. Homosexuality among men has, in fact, been legally punished much more than homosexuality among women (Tavris & Offir, 1977, p. 70).

As a consequence of these interrelated factors: low self-disclosure, competitiveness, homophobia and other issues, many men feel surprisingly lonely. They can identify with the factory employee interviewed in the documentary "Men's Lives" who said, "A man is lucky if he has one good friend."

Often for a man the only emotional link is with a woman. Pleck (1977, pp. 3–4) says, "In traditional male/female relationships, men experience their emotions vicariously through women. Many men have learned to depend on women to help them express their emotions for them. At an ultimate level, many men are unable to feel emotionally alive except through relationships with women."

When that linkage is severed the effect on the man may be severe. Divorce, death of a wife, or ending an affair are times when a man's need for emotional care and dependency are often first noticed by him. For the male seemingly in control, unneedy and invulnerable, the emotional pain is often a surprise. Such men often cannot ask for help from friends, relatives, or community care-givers because that would be showing weakness.

Research suggests that men have a harder time than women when affairs end (Hill, Rubin, & Peplau, 1976). In a study cited by Bloom, Asher, and White (1978) admission rates to mental hospitals consistently show this to be true in terms of marriages. Males with disrupted marriages have rates that are nine times greater than those for males with undisrupted marriages (30.0 versus 3.3 per 1,000). For females the differential also exists but is only three times greater (10.7 versus 3.2 per 1,000). Bloom, Asher, and White (1978) conclude:

> In general, then the relationship between marital disruption and psychopathology appears to be stronger for men than for women. There is an incongruity between this general finding and the commonly held belief that marital disruption is usually a far more difficult problem for women [p. 871].

The male liberationists are trying to teach men to develop emotional friendships with each other. In the meantime, men often cope with these situations by driving fast, drinking, fighting, engaging in a flurry of casual sex, playing pinball and, for professional men, working harder.

4. *Vocational Success is Everything*

The last problem area we will consider is the supremacy of work and career success. Whereas adult women are often skewered by the ambivalence of the career/homemaker conflict (Farmer, 1976), adult males see a clear path. The path leads to the world of work where there is only one game. That game is king of the hill. The narrow success-at-all-costs funnel for adult males is currently being questioned and criticized by behavioral science researchers.

For men occupational success accounts for most of the self-esteem variance (Morgan, Skovholt, & Orr, 1978). Even the obituaries remind the relatives of a man's occupation. They often state: John Smith, bricklayer, teacher, manager of . . . . And the first question from the stranger after the introduction is "What do you do?" Tavris and Offir (1977, p. 220) state "wives have alternatives to work that men do not. A man without a job and a woman without a husband each lack the key ingredient to their respective identites. They are, some might say, like a meal without wine or a day without sunshine."

Since getting to the top of the hill is the way to go and it is a long climb, men often devote themselves entirely to their job. Such devotion entails a high degree of selfishness because work demands must come first (Tavris & Offir, 1977).

Professional men who spend their time as workaholics, to use a popular term, suffer from an assortment of problems. For example, Sheehy (1976) in *Passages* discusses how men push the career accelerator to the floor in their 20s and 30s while their children want fathers around to play and talk with. When in their 40s the men finally want to involve themselves with their children, it is often too late. The children have become teenagers and are uprooting themselves and leaving home.

Work success often does not bring with it the expected satisfaction. One corporate man said, in looking back after thirty-five years in business, that the predominant thing was fear. They might be winning; you might be losing (Maccoby, 1976, p. 189). Unfortunately, in king of the hill there is only one winner. This is why often supposedly successful men feel like failures. They did not get to the very top.

Another problem for professional men concerns retirement time. When most of the self-esteem variance comes from occupational success, retirement must of necessity be a hazardous time. The role strain at retirement time is more kind to homemaking women, for those women continue their roles and maintain their positions while their men lose their power and importance.

The real losers at the king of the hill, however, are not the professional men who struggle with workaholicism, "finding psychic rewards," reaching the top, arranging schedules with a working wife, or other higher-order concerns. The real losers are the men who are at the bottom of the hill looking straight up. Included here are teenage inner-city males and long-term marginal male workers.

Although occupational success is the plum for all men in the society, inner-city minority teenage males have little chance to succeed at king of the hill. Borow (Note 3) expresses this pessimism when he writes:

> The dismal social consequences of maladaptive behavior among the victims of psychosocial deprivation can often be clearly seen in relation to the work role. Even in an age of affluence with its changing meanings of work, learning how to make the transition to worker remains a focal developmental task for the majority of American adolescents. The formidable array of conditions which make rational choice, planning and adjustment difficult for large numbers of today's middle- and upper-class youth—prolonged economic dependence through adolescence, delayed entrance into the labor force, heightened formal educational barriers to work entry, the paucity of visible occupational role models, the impersonality and enormous complexity of the contemporary technical work structure, the rapid rate of occupational innovation and obsolescence—all of these combine to produce a particularly disastrous effect for many among the severely disadvantaged.

These young males with unemployment rates six times the national average suffer from persistent feelings of inadequacy, a lack of adequate career planning, a chasm between the dream job and reality, premature occupational foreclosure, and a lack of competence in moving through the credentialing maze (Himes, 1964; Borow, Note 3).

When considering these young males it does not seem too speculative to spin a series of correlations between (1) the lack of viable routes to entering king of the hill, (2) the stereotypic male translation of hopelessness and despair into rage and violence, and (3) the end result—murder as the leading cause of death for nonwhite young males (Rushforth et. al, 1977). A second group who suffer are the marginal male workers, the "long-term losers who have been repeatedly clobbered and see themselves as inadequate male figures . . . and reek self-contempt" (Borow, Note 4).

The theory of learned helplessness (Seligman, Klein, & Miller, 1976) can be used to explain the behavior of these men. One of the central ways these men deal with the dehumanization they experience from work is to somatize their despair. Pain clinics and rehabilitation units that specialize in psychological approaches to chronic pain and disability usually find that their male patients have work histories that are barren of rewards. The Social Security Administration's Bureau of Hearings and Appeals regularly adjudicates the cases of large numbers of men who see themselves as inadequate males and workers and who seek an unconscious escape from the further prospect of dehumanizing work through claiming physical disabilities (Borow, Note 4).

"Measuring masculinity by the size of the paycheck" (Gould, 1976) is a reality that is a two-edged sword. For many men the world of work offers a rich variety of privileges. For others, forced to play king of the hill because there are no options, the costs are very high.

In summary, what we have just done is review selective problem areas that exist for men in the present system—the early school experience, restrictive emotionality, and the emphasis on first aggression and then work success. The recognition of these troublespots and their consequences sustains the growing male involvement in alternatives to traditional sexual and gender behavior and norms.

UNDERLYING TRENDS SUPPORTING CHANGE

The analysis of causes for change has been restricted so far to the immediate reasons why men and women might feel impelled to work for change. We cannot assume that these immediate reasons of self-interest are the only causal agents underlying the sociocultural changes.

In the authors' view the changes and readjustments in the lives of men and women are also a function of underlying ecological, ideological, and technological trends. These trends are affecting our lives in many ways other than the sexual assignment of tasks and attributes, but their summary influence on sexuality and gender needs to be made explicit.

Some of these trends are worldwide; others are peculiar to the highly urbanized, industrialized, and wealthy populations of the world. Some of the trends receive much public attention, and their effects are widely discussed and debated. One example is ecological (mankind and environment), in particular focusing on overpopulation and limited natural resources. Another example is ideological, the egalitarian philosophies and movements. Other underlying trends are less publicized. The technological trends that require less physical strength and more skill and sophistication diminish the relevance of traditional divisions of labor by gender. Corresponding advances in death-dealing technology are linked with increasingly negative evaluations of some traditional masculine character traits.

1. Ecological Trends

World population growth and an increasing public awareness of the limits of many natural resources are related to the changes in gender roles. The population issue has most directly affected women, while the resource question and its economic consequences confront both men and women.

The ability to reproduce other human beings is essential to the species and has been highly valued in all human societies. Although both sexes are necessary, the reproductive capacity of women has been especially treasured as one of their most valuable attributes, and bearing and rearing children have been considered among women's natural and vital responsibilities.

Fathering in our society, as in many others, has traditionally occupied much less of men's time and energy than mothering has for women. The preparation for parenting responsibilities has been central in the socialization of girls and women, and pregnancy and child rearing have occupied large blocks of time for many adult women. Mothering and grandmothering were women's traditional careers in our society, and the home was their workplace.

With dramatic increases in health care and world population, overpopulation rather than underpopulation is now seen by many people as the peril. Popular values are shifting so that fecundity is now more negatively than positively valued. These changes in values coincide with more efficient technological modes of birth control (both contraception and abortion). Now many children are often seen not as a blessing, but rather as an economic drain on the family and a threat to the survival and progress of our species and society. Improved nutrition and health care have greatly increased the likelihood of a child's survival, and parenting strategies have been changing from one of safety in numbers to one of greater investment in fewer children.

A further factor is the lengthening life span. The post-menopausal phase of women's lives is longer, but young American women in the 1950's, 1960's and 1970's have not been prepared for this second half of their adult lives (LeFevre 1973). Young women have focused on preparation for the carrying out of the mother role. What do these women do from age fifty to eighty? The mothering is done, and the children have grown and gone away. When the life expectancy was less and childbearing more frequent and more hazardous, this was not such a problem.

The birthrate decreases; mothering becomes less anticipated and less highly valued, and the life span increases. Relatively less time in a person's life is spent preparing for and raising children. Many young people today do not anticipate having any children, and there are numerous married couples who remain without children by preference. Their time and energy are released from parenting for other purposes.

People use that time and energy for both recreation and work, responding to both the pleasure principle and the work ethic. There is a noticeable increase in the U.S.A. in recreational participation, with men and women going on more vacations and devoting more attention and resources to sports, games, exercises, and other amusements. This increased recreation coincides with, and is often financed by, more people working.

A disproportionate percentage of these new workers are women. Women are more tied than men to preparing for, bearing, and rearing children. As these expectations and responsibilities decline, adult women shift their energies into work avenues, and girls prepare for outside the home employment and self-actualization through careers rather than through mothering.

The trends toward working women and two paycheck families are also supported by national and world inflationary trends. Inflation and the work ethic result in an increasing work orientation for women outside the home, and this, in turn, supports the demands for equal treatment in the workplace.

Although more dramatic in some places and at certain times, inflation is a worldwide trend. Both ecological and economic elements contribute to it. Usually inflation is treated as an economic matter influenced by market conditions and government policies. Demand for a product exceeds its supply, so the producers and suppliers raise the price. This concise explanation glosses over the significance of ecoloical and cultural elements that help determine the supply and the demand.

A larger world population obviously increases the demand, but two important concepts need to be understood to more fully appreciate the ecological aspect. The concepts are limiting factors and absolute scarcity. Any organism (or system) depends on a number of elements for its survival. The factor or factors in shortest supply are the ones that limit the organism's (or system's) survival and development. These may be in short supply because the price is not right, in which case it is an economic relationship of supply, demand, and price. Or the factors may be unavailable because there simply are no more of them; they are finite, and the limits have been reached. In this latter case it is an ecological relationship of limiting factors and absolute scarcity.

We all have become increasingly aware of the finite nature of a number of limiting factors, most spectacularly petroleum. This awareness is expressed politically and economically by the increased importance of oil-producing countries and the increased prices and insecurity of oil and, inevitably, all oil-based products and services.

The cultural aspect of inflation relates to the demand for goods and services. There are essentially three options when something becomes more expensive. One is to tighten the belt and do without. Another is to substitute something else that is cheaper. Both of these two responses lessen the demand. The third option is to pay the price, whatever it is. Paying the price maintains demand.

Choosing one option or another depends, among other things, on people's values and standards. The American society is consumer-oriented (see Ideological Trends below), and Americans have responded to inflation by seeking more money to satisfy their customary demands. One consequence is that wives and mothers have gone to work in income-producing jobs so that they and their families may continue to enjoy their accustomed standard of living.

Even if husbands were opposed to their wives working, the material advantage of two paychecks in a time of rising prices is a potent advocate for working women. Attention has been focused on the threat that working women pose to working men, but many men support working women because these women are their wives. The women are bringing home the eggs while the men are bringing home the bacon. Or, instead of using a subsistence example, a more realistic case for many people is that the two paychecks combined allow the family to buy all that it is used to—and more—so they may continue the pursuit of the American material dream.

2. Ideological Trends

Dreams are important. Changes in men's and women's roles cannot be thought of as simply consequences of the number of people in the world, the quantities of natural resources, or the prices of commodities. These statistics are absolute facts, but how the facts are perceived is also significant. People interpret those facts today as meaning overpopulation, scarcity, and inflation.

Perceptions are social facts. They form the basis for decisions in an ideological climate that predisposes people to choose in certain ways. Prices rise, and people choose to do without or to work harder. Perceptions and choices express people's values, their beliefs about what should and should not be, and their rankings of certain events as more desirable than others.

Values and beliefs also influence the current shifts in sexual and gender behavior. It is not our intent to conduct in this article a profound analysis of American ideology. It is important, however, to mention certain principles that seem most relevant to a discussion of sexual and gender behavior.

The three principles that appear most directly related are *egalitarianism, individualism,* and *materialism.* Egalitarianism is the most obvious and the most discussed.[4] Equal opportunities and equal rights are seen as the central ideal in the worldwide trend toward sexual, racial, and religious change. This trend is evident in the fracturing of empires through the anticolonial movement and the numerous wars of liberation—each people asserting its right to equal recognition and respect.

In the U.S.A. egalitarianism is strongly linked with individualism and materialism. The direction of social change is a synthesis of the three principles. In the U.S.A. the most important social unit is the individual, not the group or society, and the goals toward which individuals strive are often material ones. One example of this is the popular expression, "If you're so smart why aren't you rich?"

In consequence, the movement in the U.S.A. is primarily toward equal rights for the individual as a wage-earner and consumer. The major changes concern the opportunities and conditions in education (that equips people for better employment), employment, and consumption.

The fundamental complexes of values (egalitarianism, individualism, and materialism) have always been part of the American national culture, as evidenced by de Tocqueville in his volumes of *Democracy in America* that were first published in 1835 and 1840. They co-existed, however, with slavery and the concept of women as chattel or property of their fathers and husbands.

The evolution of American society since then has been a gradual one with several memorable watersheds: emancipation, women's suffrage, and desegregation. At each transition there was a redefinition of human rights and a redistribution of political power.

The major changes have not consisted of eliminating or substituting one principle for another. The changes have primarily served to redefine the application of the existing principles, that is, to decide to whom or to what categories of people the principles apply. In the early years of the American republic the principles applied to Caucasian men only. Gradually the boundaries of the privileged category have been extended to include more and more people. Of most relevance here is the inclusion of women.

Both men and women generally adhere to their national ideology. The ideological principles channel the ambitions and directions of reformers and sustain their arguments because the audience shares allegiance to the same principles. The clearer the moral argument, the more irresistible it is to both sexes.

---

[4]In the U.S.A. equality of opportunity is stressed but inequality of wealth and position has always been accepted and positively valued if it represents (or is seen to represent) the reward for individual achievement. There is a strengthening countercurrent against even these inequalities.

It is important to point out here that both men and women oppose the movement toward sexual equality, and both men and women support it. The two sides are not sexually homogeneous and opposed. An important reason why more men and women do not now support the movement is because the clear moral argument is buried in a confusion of other more debatable issues of style, personal preference, marriage, and family life.

3. Technological Trends

Ideological arguments for equal access to and treatment in the workplace are reinforced by two technological trends in urban industrialized societies. One trend is a widespread devaluation of physical strength in favor of educated skills. Skills, not strength, have become essential for performance and success. Another trend is the significant increase, both at work and at home, in the level of required skills. Both men and women have become more skilled at and accustomed to a machine-aided, technologically more complex environment. These trends, in conjunction with the demographic change toward fewer or no children, diminish the physical and social rational for the traditional sexual division of labor.

In urban industrialized societies physical strength is relatively insignificant as a work requirement (Gagnon, 1976). Both authors were struck by this point when we were co-teaching a course on masculinity and male roles. In the class there were three college scholarship football players, defensive and offensive linesmen. Beyond the requirements of professional sports that consume the energy of relatively few men, we could think of few occupational avenues for these men where they could use their tremendous upper body strength.

Can you think of many jobs with the big three—money, power, and status—that demand tremendous physical strength? Certainly there are many jobs that demand strength in which male workers predominate—for example; miner, construction worker, some factory employment. The higher status positions, however, of physician, attorney, captain of industry, professor, and our most essential warriors—missile operator and pilot—seldom demand that one bench press anything!

John Henry and Paul Bunyan are archaic figures because few American men now devote their lives to physical labor (Steinman & Foxe, 1974, p. 5). Intellectual skills are the requirements of the modern workplace, as is evident in the increase of educated citizens from 1910 to 1970, shown by a 450% increase in college degrees (Grant & Lind, 1976), and the decrease in unskilled and farm employment from 1910 to 1970, a 200% decrease (Wolfbein, 1964). Ours is a world of offices and white collar workers.

Even under rural nonindustrial conditions the hard physical labor demands did not necessitate a sexual allocation of tasks. Although men and women differ on the basis of average body mass and strength, there is more variation within each sexual population than there is a difference between them.

The natural potential for sexual differences in body mass and strength is exaggerated by social and cultural factors. A cultural attribution of strength and aggression to men has been an important factor in maintaining sexual distinctions. Men in many societies cultivate their strength and work to develop it, while many women do not. Although no longer important vocationally, strength continues to be psychologically important to most men.

The flourishing sports and recreational activities of the 1970s are an artificial means we have developed to keep our bodies in use in ways that formerly were natural. Imagine trying to explain our health problems related to obesity and the difficulties of getting enough exercise to an adult (man or woman) who lives by the sweat of his or her brow.

Gagnon (1976) is right when he says physical strength has lost its essential significance in dividing the work of men and women. It is important to note that the resultant change is gradual. The notion of a socialization lag is one way to understand the continuing validation of a gender role attribute that is gradually going the way of the big American car. In industrial nations men and women continue to define physical ability as a highly prized male attribute. Examples from the U.S.A. include winning at arm wrestling, ringing the bell at the county fair (as depicted in the documentary film ''Men's lives''), and quickly opening the family food jars that the women cannot open.

Concomitant with the devaluation of strength is an increase in needed machine- and industry-related skills. Both at home and at work a person needs to learn and adapt to new technologies. The more significant change is at home because the increased technological complexity there diminishes the previous disparity between traditional household labors and innovative office work.

When you look at the instruction manual for a microwave oven you realize that it was written for a technologically aware audience. A more general example concerns laundry. The combination of types of fabrics, each with its own washing, drying, and ironing instructions, and types of soaps, detergents, bleaches, softeners, and so forth, makes an industrial experience out of every trip to the laundry room.

Home and office have converged in terms of the skills and background a person needs to work in either. There is little technological difference between a push-button job and a pop-in dinner. Both involve some mechanical manipulation of highly processed inputs. Neither involve traditional skills or physical strength. Both actions (pushing buttons and popping dinners) share a character that is culturally neither masculine nor feminine.

Technological innovations in household tasks have not only changed the character of housework and the qualifications of housewives, thus supporting the emergence of working women; the innovations have also greatly increased the viability of single living and single parenting. Of particular importance in this regard are processed and semiprocessed foods, microwave ovens, and clothes that do not need ironing.

A division of labor in which one person works to provide money and another works to maintain and operate the home is still attractive to many people. Whatever the sex of either worker, the division and coordination of labor eases the pressure on both. Increasingly, however, more people are living alone and more adults are living as single parents. This trend is facilitated by the speed and ease with which meals may be prepared and clothes processed.

The trend, in turn, influences the allocation and modeling of traditionally sex-specific behavior patterns. A single person or parent of whichever sex occupies almost all of the roles and peforms almost all of the functions that a couple would traditionally.

In addition to the effects already mentioned, there is one last way in which a technological trend is related to rethinking gender characteristics, this time particularly a male one. Death technology is well-developed and well-financed. In order to make future hosts of future wars feel better we even have clean bombs that save the real estate. The increasing range and power of death technology and the increasing speed with which nations (and those individuals with their fingers on the buttons) can respond to provocations make widespread destruction more probable. Many people are aware and afraid of this probability.

One consequence of the technology and fear is a devaluation of intemperate aggression. Just as the pattern of adolescent aggression may have unfortunate effects on many young men, that same pattern may be lethal for many people when displayed by political or military leaders.

People now are more reluctant to be represented politically by men who like to practice confrontation diplomacy or who impulsively "shoot from the hip." Those character and behavior patterns were perhaps appropriate on the frontiers in the past, but the human species cannot afford any more the sort of mistakes to which those patterns are liable. The world is too vulnerable now.

THE POSSIBILITY AND DESIRABILITY OF CHANGE

This evaluation of male aggression, and indeed the entire process of sociocultural change documented in this article, rests on a key assumption that changes can be made in the character traits and behavior patterns traditionally attributed to men and women. The assumption involves the hypothesis that these traits and activities are overwhelmingly determined by society rather than genetics.

Ethnographic studies support this hypothesis (Beach 1977; Ford & Beach 1951; Friedl 1975). All societies have made distinctions between the sexes but the specific distinctions have differed from one culture to another. Sometimes men are described as A, women as B. Sometimes men are described as C, women as D, and sometimes men and women share large chunks of E and F. The plasticity of gender has enabled societies to demand different attributes and behaviors from the sexes at different times and to maximize biological differences or to minimize them.

Of particular importance to men's lives today is the suggestion by anthropologist Marvin Harris that male supremacy is on the way out in all industrialized nations. He says that it was just a phase in the evolution of culture (Tavris, 1975). Contemporary psychological theory and practice agree with this view, and the new sexual research endorses a number of ideas that contradict old beliefs.

New research suggests that, apart from obvious physiological differences, the sexes are more alike than different. Even the physiology of the sexes is now seen as more similar. Researchers find that hormonal cycling and the sexual response cycle turn out to be surprisingly alike for men and women (Saxton, 1977, p. 72).

New research points to the biological primacy of females. Woman comes out of Adam's rib? No. All fetuses will become female unless at four points during prenatal development specific inputs and responses occur. Only then will the fetus become male. Money and Tucker (1975, p. 48) consider each of these points a critical junction because male development hinges on the results. The four crucial events involve sex chromosomes and hormones and the development of the gonads, the internal and the external genitalia.

There seem to be very few psychological sex differences, and those are averages. As was noted above concerning body mass and strength, the variation within each sexual population is greater than the mean difference between the two. Of sexual comparisons the most cited mean differences have been in visual spacial abilities, verbal abilities, quantitative abilities, and aggression (Tavris & Offir, 1977, p. 33).

Consider the trait of nurturance. We think that women are more loving toward children than men but research lends little support to such a common belief. Infants bring out the same "ecstacy response" in males and females. Females express it more in public, but men also experience it (Tavris & Offir, 1977, p. 52).

These anthropological, physiological, and psychological findings support the assumption that gender roles and assignments of character traits can be changed. Other research addresses the question of whether, and in what ways, the changes are beneficial or not.

In terms of character traits, the new psychological code word for mental health is androgyny, the possession of both male- and female-associated traits.[5] Research shows that people of either sex in this society are interpersonally most competent if they possess stereotyped male and

[5]It is noteworthy that androgyny as an outcome has been thoughtfully criticized by Sampson (1977).

female traits such as toughness and tenderness, resistance to pressure, and nurturance, achievement, and affiliation (Bem, 1975a).

What is the impact of working mothers on their children? The earlier view of maternal employment was that such work adversely affected the children. The new gender role research questions this view. A well respected recent critique suggests that the effects of maternal employment on children is a complex question requiring sophisticated research (Hoffman, 1974).

As a role model, according to Hoffman, the working mother has children who have less traditional sex role concepts, have higher evaluations of female competence and seemingly are psychologically healthier. What are the effects of the mother's emotional state on children? Hoffman says if the mother enjoys her work, if the homemaker versus career role strain is only moderate and if one does not feel overly guilty about work, then children will probably do well.

What are the childrearing practices of working mothers? Hoffman says fathers are more involved with child rearing and this is positive for both male and female children. These children are high in independence training and have more household responsibilities. Concerning supervision, Hoffman says working mothers provide less adequate supervision for their children, but there is little empirical information about maternal deprivation.

Overall, Hoffman is positive about the effects of maternal employment on children, but notes that the meaning maternal employment has for the family and the social setting will detemine the effects.

Affectionate fathering is now coming into style like frozen yogurt, mopeds, jogging, and cross country skiing. And it is not any too soon, according to some new research that reveals that fathers average only 12 minutes per day with their children (Tavris & Offir, 1977, p. 232). This is related to the adult male focus on work and career that was previously discussed. The minor involvement that fathers traditionally have with children is unfortunate because fathers are now seen to be important to their children's social and emotional development (Biller & Meredith, 1974; Lamb, 1976; Lynn, 1974).

Some years ago Margaret Mead suggested that fathers were a biological necessity while being a social accident. Present research disagrees. Parke and Sawin (1977), authors of an article "Fathering: It's a major role," say:

> Our studies of fathers confirm that they are not a social accident at all. They contribute significantly to an infant's social and intellectual growth . . . . The father is not just a poor substitute for the mother, he makes his own unique contributions to the care and development of infants and young children [p. 109].

Other current child development articles have such tradition-defying titles as Earls' (1976) article, "The fathers (not the mothers): Their importance and influence with infants and young children." Earls (1976, p. 220) says: "the research . . . represents an impressive body of findings that paternal loss or deprivation is an important contributing factor in later maladjustment, especially for boys."

It is important to note, however, that affectionate fathering of young children is more an idea than a reality at this time. This is consistent with our earlier statement that women have been changing more than men.

MALE REACTIONS

What are men's reactions to these changes? How are men responding to the pressures to accommodate and the injunctions to become androgynous, substitute affection for aggression, and divert some of their time and energy from work to human relationships?

Men seem to have a less difficult time with current gender role issues than women. Many men feel only minimum gender role strain (Deutsch & Gilbert, 1976; Komarovsky, 1976, p. 9). Women, on the other hand, are faced with major retooling in moving away from reproduction as the essential task of adult life.

Although men experience less direct effect, they are intensely involved with the effects on women's lives because men and women live together. Sociologist Michael Schwartz (Note 5) notes that the analogies between feminism and the civil rights movement miss one essential: Blacks and Whites do not live in the same intensely personal relationships that are true of men and women.

There is an ecological balance between men and women. When one changes, the other must also change. A similar comparison is with the systems approach of family therapy. As one element of the family changes, other elements of necessity change too.

1. Traditional Men

In *The longest war: Sex differences in perspective,* Tavris and Offir (1977, p. 9) ask, "Why have men had so few fantasies of an intellectual partner, an equal, a friend?"

Traditional men define the roles of men and women very differently. The sexual scheme is one of opposites. These men define themselves as that which women are not. Men do what women do not, and masculinity is that which femininity is not. The loss of traditional distinctions is, of course, disturbing and unwelcome. It is a direct threat to their identity.

These men see femininity as based on biology. Women have natural and valuable roles as mothers. Men are less necessary in this regard with no clear role: "since one male is physically capable of inseminating many females, a high survival rate for the male is of little consequence to the species" (Etkin, 1967, p. 71).

The male identity then focuses on the defense of women and children and the provision of food and shelter. Men are soldiers and hunters, keeping the wolf away and bringing home the bacon. These activities and responsibilities provide a clear guide and justification for their lives.

Today women are entering the hunting, fishing, and fighting arenas. At one midwestern university the increase in female students in the professional schools of medicine, law, and business was 330%, 550%, and 450%, respectively, from 1960 to 1976 (Hutter, 1978). Traditional men sense only increased competition with no new options for themselves.

Their ideas about the sexes are based on a pattern of oppositions. These men are uncomfortable sharing occupations and positions with women. Other choices such as fewer work responsibilities and more child care opportunities are not enticing for the same reason. Certainly house-husbanding is not a viable option.

The increased competition in work is discomforting for another reason, also. Traditionally when women have entered a career field the field's status has gradually fallen: clerical work here, medicine in Russia (Tavris & Offir, 1977, p. 16). These men sense no advantages in gender role realignments.

2. Men in Transition

Men in transition are trying to escape the traps of traditional men that Myron Brenton (1966) describes:

> As long as men feel that the equality of women will emasculate them, it is exactly what will happen. As long as men identify themselves so narrowly with the bread-winning role, with the competitive demands of their consumer society, with narrow and noncreative work, their psychic equilibrium will be shaky [p. 203].

Men in transition have developed a sensitivity to the dilemmas of contemporary women and believe the women they love and cherish must have better options. These men read the popular feminist literature and are offended not so much by the attacks upon men as by the limits they sense for women. These men react to the dead ends that women often face in traditional roles. These men know, along with Rollo May (1972), that powerlessness leads to madness or to one of its minor forms, such as living vicariously through one's husband. "We work for Texaco." "The Department did well this year."

These men are able, in our view, to view females in two ways: as *persons* and as *women*. Such a man can work for a female supervisor because he can see her as a person. He can also feel romantic toward an achieving female because he can see her as a woman. We believe men who are comfortable with high-achieving women have developed this capacity, a cognitive capacity, to turn on and off the person/woman light bulb when interacting with a female.

Economics plays a powerful part too. Tavris and Offir (1977) say it is the economic offerings of contemporary women that give them status and power. The wages of a woman companion that amount to significantly more that "pin money" are often seen as a blessing by these men. For young college graduates the factor of two salaries often makes it possible to purchase a house. A working wife may even free a man to quit a second job, take a paternity leave, or go back to school for new training. For many husbands the two incomes make it possible to keep up with inflation, so the family may continue to satisfy its customary demands.

3. The Male Liberationists

The most direct reaction to feminism is the position of the male liberationists. Male liberation was born out of feminism. We, the authors, respond strongly to the male liberation position, but our response is both positive and negative.

Male liberationists stress the demons of masculine obsession with achievement but, in the process of focusing on overachievement, they leave a negative impression. Warren Farrell (1974) and men of similar persuasion describe men as oppressed. Here is a group of powerful, elite, suburban-reared White males, some of the most privileged people in the world, and they are complaining. These men, wringing their hands because it is hard to run the show, are described by Geng (1976) as very whiney, like colonial administrators complaining about malaria.

The abdication of responsibility that one senses from this position is noxious. It seems that male liberation, in part, emphasizes a moving away from the tough leadership positions where the solutions of psychological, social, and political problems are forged.

An ironic counterpoint, however, is that the position is in some ways even more demanding of men than traditional views of masculinity. Take, for example, race car drivers. These drivers have very traditional male personality traits (Johnsgard, 1977). The liberationists suggest that this is not enough: these men, to be fully human, must also be nurturing and affiliating.

The great gift of the male liberationists is their exploration of male socialization. Most men do not explore this, and women who explore male socialization do so as outsiders, and as outsiders who often criticize in nonconstructive ways. Male liberationists are "native explorers" or "participant observers" who are illuminating important issues and producing useful summaries of the explorations into masculinity (Ferriero, 1977).

A CONCLUDING NOTE

We, the authors, are husbands, fathers, and social scientists. One of us is a psychologist with counseling experience. The other has studied other societies as an anthropologist. Both of us have taught college courses on human sexuality and gender. We and our male friends, clients, and students are face to face with the joy, confusion, and depression that are part of normal life in this society, trying to develop and reach that "affirmation of myself" that we desire.

In the process today a number of questions arise. How are men to handle liking/loving other men? Some of our friends shake hands and punch each other. Others hug. Others are experimenting with homosexuality. How expressive should we be? How competitive? How combative?

We and many others share our lives with women. As partners and lovers we balance our ambitions and desires, our days and energies. How important are our careers and marriages to us? To them? How important should they be?

Our children are another important part of our lives. They are growing, learning, seeing us. What do we show them, tell them? How do we model the roles we want them to play? What do we want them to be? What is happening to the society that our children are growing into?

In this time of personal, social, and political uncertainty we all need to understand the interplay of forces and trends that are changing our world. One of our concerns is that one-dimensional man, the aggressive hunter/warrior, no longer fits well with our present and evolving world. In fact, one-dimensional man is one of the lethal factors in the "will the human species survive?" question.

Explorations and critiques of masculinity are especially important when we see how older male styles endanger our survival. Our world is experiencing a rapid depletion of some crucial natural resources and a simultaneous rapid increase in the human population and the technology of destruction. Our species has a history of responding to scarcities and inequalities with violence and war. Traditional male styles stress (1) the need to instill respect, (2) the readiness to meet aggression, and (3) combative ways to gain self- and other-respect. These traits are dangerous.

Justice does not come out of the barrel of a gun: death does. Our worldwide society, our Spaceship Earth, must encourage interpersonal and international styles of affiliation and merger rather than confrontation.

REFERENCE NOTES

1. Miner, R. Personal communication, March, 1978.
2. Levy, J. M. *Child and family therapy from a feminist perspective.* Children's Mental Health Unit, Shands Tecahing Hospital, University of Florida, unpublished paper, no date.
3. Borow, H. *Antecedents, concomitants, and consequences of task-oriented*

behavior in youth. Invitation paper published by the National Institute of Child Health and Human Development. Bethesda, Maryland, 1968.
4. Borow, H. Personal communication, December, 1977.
5. Schwartz, M. Personal communication, April, 1976.

REFERENCES

Alda, A. What every woman should know about men. *MS*, 1975, *4* (4), 15–16.

Baker, S. P., & Fisher, R. S. Alcohol and motorcycle fatalities. *American Journal of Public Health*, 1977, *67*, 246–249.

Balswick, J. O., & Peek, C. W. The inexpressive male. In D. S. David & R. Brannon (Eds.), *The forty-nine percent majority: The male sex role*. Reading, Mass.: Addison-Wesley, 1976.

Beach, F. A. (Ed.). *Human sexuality in four perspectives*. Baltimore: Johns Hopkins, 1977.

Bem, S. L. Sex role adaptability: One consequence of psychological androgyny. *Journal of Personality and Social Psychology*, 1975, *31*, 634–643. (a)

Bem, S. L. Androgeny vs. the tight little lives of fluffy women and chesty men. *Psychology Today*, 1975, *9* (4), 58–59, 61–62. (b)

Biller, H. B., & Meredith, D. *Father power*. New York: McKay, 1974.

Bloom, B. L., Asher, S. J., & White, S. W. Marital disruption as a stressor: A review and analysis. *Psychological Bulletin*, 1978, *85*, 867–894.

Brenton, M. *The American male*. New York: Coward-McCann, Inc., 1966.

David, D. S., & Brannon, R. (Eds.). *The forty-nine percent majority: The male sex role*. Reading, Mass.: Addison-Wesley, 1976.

Deardorff, P. A., Finch, A. J., Kendell, P. C., Lira, F., & Indrisano, V. Empathy and socialization in repeat offenders, first offenders, and normals. *Journal of Counseling Psychology*, 1975, *22*, 453–455.

Deutsch, C. J., & Gilbert, L. A. Sex role stereotypes: Effect on perceptions of self and others and on personal adjustment. *Journal of Counseling Psychology*, 1976, *23*, 373–379.

Dohrenwend, B., & Dohrenwend, B. S. Sex differences in psychiatric disorders. *American Journal of Sociology*, 1976, *81*, 1447–1459.

Dohrenwend, B., & Dohrenwend, B. S. Reply to Gove and Tudor's comment on "Sex differences in psychiatric disorders." *American Journal of Sociology*, 1977, *82*, 1336–1345.

Earls, F. The fathers (not the mothers): Their importance and influence with infants and young children. *Psychiatry*, 1976, *39*, 209–226.

Eme, R. F. Sex differences in childhood psychopathology: A review. *Psychological Bulletin*, 1979, *86*, 574–595.

Etkin, W. *Social behavior from fish to man*. Chicago: University of Chicago Press, 1967.

Farmer, H. S. What inhibits achievement and career motivation in women? *The Counseling Psychologist*, 1976, *6*(2), 12–15.

Farrell, W. *The liberated man*. New York: Bantam Books, 1974.

Fasteau, M. F. *The male machine*. New York: McGraw-Hill, 1974.

Ferriero, D. S. (Ed.). *Men's studies bibliography*. Cambridge, Mass.: Massachusetts Institute of Technology, Human Studies Collection, Humanities Library, 1977.

Ford, C. S., & Beach, F. A. *Patterns of sexual behavior.* New York: Harper & Row, 1951

Friedl, E. *Women and men: An anthropologist's view.* New York: Holt, Rinehart & Winston, 1975.

Gagnon, J. H. Physical strength, once of significance. In D. S. David & R. Brannon (Eds.), *The forty-nine percent majority: The male sex role.* Reading, Mass.: Addison-Wesley, 1976.

Geng, V. Requiem for the women's movement. *Harpers,* 1976, *253*, (1518), 49–56, 61–68.

Goldberg, H. *The hazards of being male.* New York: New American Library, 1977.

Gould, R. Measuring masculinity by the size of the paycheck. In D. S. David & R. Brannon (Eds.), *The forty-nine percent majority: The male sex role.* Reading, Mass.: Addison-Wesley, 1976.

Gove, W., & Tudor, J. Adult sex roles and mental illness. *American Journal of Sociology,* 1973, *78,* 812–835.

Gove W., & Tudor, J. Sex differences in mental illness: A comment on Dohrenwend and Dohrenwend. *American Journal of Sociology,* 1977, *82,* 1327–1336.

Grambs, J. D., & Waetjen, W. B. *Sex: Does it make a difference?* North Scituate, Mass.: Duxbury, 1975.

Grant, W. V., & Lind, C. G. *Digest of educational statistics: 1975 edition.* Washington, D.C.: U.S. Government Printing Office, 1976

Hill, C. T., Rubin, Z., & Peplau, L. A. Breakups before marriage: The end of 103 affairs. *Journal of Social Issues,* 1976, *32,* 147–168.

Himes, J. S. Some work-related cultural deprivations of lower-class Negro youth. *Journal of Marriage and the Family,* 1964, *26,* 447–449.

Hoffman, L. W. The effects of maternal employment on the child—a review of the literature. *Developmental Psychology,* 1974, *10,* 204–228.

Hutter, B. Feminist caucus issues outlined. *The Minnesota Daily,* January, 1978, p. 4.

Jeffers, R. The bloody sire. In N. Friedman & C. A. McLaughlin (Eds.), *Poetry: An introduction to its form and art.* New York: Harper, 1961.

Johnsgard, K. Personality and performance: A psychological study of amateur sports car race drivers. *Journal of Sports Medicine and Physical Fitness,* 1977, *17,* 97–104.

Jourard, S. *The transparent self.* New York: Van Nostrand, 1971.

Jourard, S. Some lethal aspects of the male role. In J. H. Pleck & J. Sawyer (Eds.), *Men and masculinity.* Englewood Cliffs, N.J.: Prentice-Hall, 1974.

Kagan, J. The child's sex role classification of school subjects. *Child Development,* 1964, *35,* 1051–1056.

Komarovsky, M. *Dilemmas of masculinity: A study of college youth.* New York: Norton, 1976.

Lamb, M. E. (Ed.). *The role of the father in child development.* New York: Wiley, 1976.

LeFevre, C. New directions for women. In E. S. Morrison & V. Borosage (Eds.), *Human sexuality: Contemporary perspectives.* Palo Alto, Calif.: National Press Books, 1973.

Lerner, I. M. *Heredity evolution and society.* San Francisco: W. H. Freeman, 1968.

Lynn, D. B. *The father: His role in child development.* Monterey, Calif.: Brooks/ Cole, 1974.

Maccoby, M. *The gamesman: The new corporate leader.* New York: Simon & Schuster, 1976.

Mandell, A. *Coming of middle age.* New York: Summit Books, 1977.

May, R. *Power and innocence.* New York: Dell, 1972.

Money, J., & Tucker, P. *Sexual signatures.* Boston: Little Brown, 1975.

Morgan, J., Skovholt, T., & Orr, J. Career counseling with men: The shifting focus. In S. Weinrach (Ed.), *Vocational counseling: Theory and techniques.* New York: McGraw-Hill, 1978.

Noblet, G. W., & Burcart, J. M. Women and crime: 1960–1970. *Social Science Quarterly,* 1976, *56*, 650–657.

Parke, R. D., & Sawin, D. B. Fathering: It's a major role. *Psychology Today,* 1977, *11* (6), 108–112.

Pleck, J. H. Men's power with women, other men, and society: A men's movement analysis. In D. Hiller & R. Sheets, (Eds.), *Women and men: The consequences of power.* Cincinnati: Office of Women's Studies, University of Cincinnati, 1977.

Rushforth, N. B., Ford, A. B., Hirsch, C. S., Rushforth, N. M., & Adelson, L. Violent death in a metropolitan county: Changing patterns in homicide (1958–1974). *New England Journal of Medicine,* 1977, *297*, 531–538.

Sampson, E. F. Psychology and the American ideal. *Journal of Personality and Social Psychology,* 1977, *35*, 767–782.

Saxton, L. *The individual, marriage, and the family.* Belmont, Calif.: Wadsworth, 1977.

Seligman, M. E. P., Klein, D. C., & Miller, W. R. Depression. In H. Leitenberg (Ed.), *Handbook of behavior modification and behavior therapy.* Englewood Cliffs, N. J.: Prentice-Hall, Inc., 1976.

Sheehy, G. *Passages.* New York: Dutton, 1976.

Statistical Abstract of the United States. Washington, D.C.: Bureau of the Census, Department of Commerce, 1976.

Steinmann, A., & Foxe, D. J. *The male dilemma: How to survive the sexual revolution.* New York: Jason Aronson, 1974.

Stockton, M. D., Edwards, D., & Hines, B. Sex offenders: Clinical characteristics and treatment methods. In T. M. Skovholt, P. G. Schauble, & R. Davis (Eds.), *Counseling men.* Monterey, Calif.: Brooks/Cole, 1980.

Tavris, C. Male supremacy is on the way out. It was just a phase in the evolution of culture. A conversation with Marvin Harris. *Psychology Today,* 1975, *8* (8), 61–69.

Tavris, C., & Offir, C. *The longest war: Sex differences in perspective.* New York: Harcourt Brace Jovanovich, 1977.

Tooley, K. M. 'Johnny, I hardly knew ye': Toward revision of the theory of male psychosexual development. *American Journal of Orthopsychiatry,* 1977, *47*, 184–195.

Werry, J. S., & Quay, H. C. The prevalence of behavior symptoms in younger elementary school children. *American Journal of Orthopsychiatry,* 1971, *41*, 136–143.

Wolfbein, S. L. Labor trends, manpower, and automation. In H. Borow (Ed.), *Man in a world at work.* Boston: Houghton Mifflin, 1964.

THEORETICAL ARTICLES 2

Men's Power with Women, Other Men, and Society: A Men's Movement Analysis

JOSEPH H. PLECK
Institute for Social Research
University of Michigan*

My aim in this paper is to analyze men's power from the perspective afforded by the emerging antisexist men's movement. In the last several years, an antisexist men's movement has appeared in North America and in the Western European countries. While it is not so widely known as the women's movement, the men's movement has generated a variety of books, publications, and organizations (David & Brannon, 1975; Farrell, 1975; Fasteau, 1974; Nichols, 1975; Petras, 1975; Pleck & Sawyer, 1974)[1] and is now an established presence on the sex role scene. The present and future political relationship between the women's movement and the men's movement raises complex questions that I do not deal with here, though they are clearly important ones. Instead, here I present my own view of the contribution that the men's movement and the men's analysis make to a

"Men's Power With Women, Other Men and Society: A Men's Movement Analysis," by J. H. Pleck. In D. V. Hiller and R. Sheets (Eds.), *Women and Men: The Consequences of Power*. Reprinted by permission of the author.
    *Now at Wellesley College

feminist understanding of men and power, and of power relations between the sexes. First, I will analyze men's power over women, particularly in relation to the power that men often perceive women have over them. Then I will analyze two other power relationships men are implicated in—men's power with other men, and men's power in society more generally—and suggest how these two other power relationships interact with men's power over women.

MEN'S POWER OVER WOMEN, AND WOMEN'S POWER OVER MEN

It is becoming increasingly recognized that one of the most fundamental questions raised by the women's movement is not a question about women at all, but rather a question about men: why do men oppress women? There are two general kinds of answers to this question. The first is that men want power over women because it is in their rational self-interest to do so, to have the concrete benefits and privileges that power over women provides them. Having power, it is rational to want to keep it. The second kind of answer is that men want to have power over women because of deep-lying psychological needs in the male personality. These two views are not mutually exclusive, and there is certainly ample evidence for both. The final analysis of men's oppression of women will have to give attention equally to its rational and irrational sources.

I will concentrate my attention here on the psychological sources of men's needs for power over women. Let us consider first the most common and common-sense psychological analysis of men's need to dominate women, which takes as its starting point the male child's early experience with women. The male child, the argument goes, perceives his mother and his predominantly female elementary school teachers as dominating and controlling. These relationships *do* in reality contain elements of domination and control, probably exacerbated by the restriction of women's opportunities to exercise power in most other areas. As a result, men feel a lifelong psychological need to free themselves from or prevent their domination by women. The argument is, in effect, that men oppress women as adults because they experienced women as oppressing them as children.

According to this analysis, this process operates in a vicious circle. In each generation, adult men restrict women from having power in almost all domains of social life except childrearing. As a result, male children feel powerless and dominated, grow up needing to restrict women's power, and thus the cycle repeats itself. It follows from this analysis that the way to break this vicious circle is to make it possible for women to exercise power outside of parenting and parent-like roles, and to get men to do their half share of parenting.

There may be a kernel of truth in this "mother domination" theory of sexism for some men, and the social changes in the organization of child care that this theory suggests are certainly desirable. As a general explanation of men's needs to dominate women, however, this theory has been quite overworked. This theory holds women themselves, rather than men, ultimately responsible for the oppression of women—in William Ryan's phrase, "blaming the victims" of oppression for their own oppression (Ryan, 1970). The recent film *One Flew Over the Cuckoo's Nest* presents an extreme example of how women's supposed domination of men is used to justify sexism. This film portrays the archetypal struggle between a female figure depicted as domineering and castrating, and a rebellious male hero (played by Jack Nicholson) who refuses to be emasculated by her. This struggle escalates to a climatic scene in which Nicholson throws her on the floor and nearly strangles her to death—a scene that was accompanied by wild cheering from the audience that I saw the film with. For this performance, Jack Nicholson won the Academy Award as the best actor of the year, an indication of how successful the film is in seducing its audience to accept this act of sexual violence as legitimate and even heroic. The hidden moral message of the film is that because women dominate men, the most extreme forms of sexual violence are not only permissible for men but indeed are morally obligatory.

To account for men's needs for power over women, it is ultimately more useful to examine some other ways that men feel women have power over them than fear of maternal domination.[2] There are two forms of power that men perceive women as holding over them that derive more directly from traditional definitions of adult male and female roles and that have implications that are far more compatible with a feminist perspective.

The first power that men perceive women having over them is *expressive power,* the power to express emotions. It is well known that in traditional male/female relationships, women are supposed to express their needs for achievement only vicariously through the achievements of men. It is not so widely recognized, however, that this dependency of women on men's achievement has a converse. In traditional male/female relationships, men experience their emotions vicariously through women. Many men have learned to depend on women to help them express their emotions, indeed to express their emotions for them. At an ultimate level, many men are unable to feel emotionally alive except through relationships with women. A particularly dramatic example occurs in an earlier Jack Nicholson film, *Carnal Knowledge.* Art Garfunkel, at one point early in his romance with Candy Bergen, tells Nicholson that she makes him aware of thoughts he "never even knew he had." Although Nicholson is sleeping with Bergen and Garfunkel is not, Nicholson feels tremendously deprived in comparison when he hears this. In a dramatic scene, Nicholson then goes to her and angrily demands: "You tell him his thoughts, now you tell me *my* thoughts!" When women withhold and refuse to exercise this expressive power for men's benefit, many men, like Nicholson, feel abject and try all the harder to get women to play their traditional expressive role.

A second form of power that men attribute to women is *masculinity-validating* power. In traditional masculinity, to experience oneself as masculine requires that women play their prescribed role of doing the things that make men feel masculine. Another scene from *Carnal Knowledge* provides a pointed illustration. In the closing scene of the movie, Nicholson has hired a call girl whom he has rehearsed and coached in a script telling him how strong and manly he is, in order to get him sexually aroused. Nicholson seems to be in control, but when she makes a mistake in her role, his desperate reprimands show just how dependent he is on her playing out the masculinity-validating script he has created. It is clear that what he is looking for in this encounter is not so much sexual gratification as it is validation of himself as a man—which only women can give him. As with women's expressive power, when women refuse to exercise their masculinity-validating power for men, many men feel lost and bereft, and frantically attempt to force women back into their accustomed role.

As I suggested before, men's need for power over women derives from both men's pragmatic self-interest and from men's psychological needs. It would be a mistake to overemphasize men's psychological needs as the sources of men's needs to control women, in comparison with simple rational self-interest. But if we are looking for the psychological sources of men's needs for power over women, men's perception that women have expressive power and masculinity-validating power over them is critical to analyze. These are the two powers men perceive women as having, which they fear women will no longer exercise in their favor. These are the two resources women possess that men fear women will withold, and whose threatened or actual loss leads men to such frantic attempts to reassert power over women.

Men's dependence on women's power to express men's emotions and to validate men's masculinity have placed heavy burdens on women. By and large, these are not powers over men that women have wanted to hold. These are powers over men that men have themselves handed over to women, by defining the male role as being emotionally cool and inexpressive, and as being ultimately validated by heterosexual success.

There is reason to think that over the course of recent history—as male/male friendship has declined, and as dating and marriage have occurred more universally and at younger ages—the demands on men to be emotionally inexpressive and to prove masculinity through relating to women have become stronger. As a result, men have given women increasingly more expressive power and more masculinity-validating power over them, and have become increasingly dependent on women for emotional and sex role validation. In the context of this increased dependency on women's power, the emergence of the women's movement now, with women asserting their right not to play these roles for men, has hit men with a special force.

It is in this context that the men's movement and men's groups place so much emphasis on men learning to express and experience their emotions with each other, and learning how to validate themselves and each other as persons, instead of needing women to validate them emotionally and as men. When men realize that they can develop in themselves the power to experience themselves emotionally and to validate themselves as persons, they will not feel the dependency on women for these essential needs that has led in the past to so much male fear, resentment, and need to control women. Then men will be emotionally more free to negotiate the pragmatic realignment of power between the sexes that is underway in our society.

MEN'S POWER WITH OTHER MEN

After considering men's power over women in relation to the power men perceive women having over them, let us consider men's power over women in a second context: the context of men's power relationships with other men. In recent years, we have come to understand that relations between men and women are governed by a sexual politics that exists outside individual men's and women's needs and choices. It has taken us much longer to recognize that there is a systematic sexual politics of male/male relationships as well. Under patriarchy, men's relationships with other men cannot help but be shaped and patterned by patriarchal norms, though they are less obvious than the norms governing male/female relationships. A society could not have the kinds of power dynamics that exist between women and men in our society without certain kinds of systematic power dynamics operating among men as well.

One dramatic example illustrating this connection occurs in the recent novel *Small Changes* (Piercy, 1978). In a flashback scene, a male character goes along with several friends to gang-rape a woman. When his turn comes, he is impotent, whereupon the other men grab him, pulling his pants down to rape *him*. This scene powerfully conveys one form of the relationship between male/female and male/male sexual politics. The point is that men do not just happily bond together to oppress women. In addition to hierarchy over women, men create hierarchies and rankings among themselves according to criteria of "masculinity." Men at each rank of masculinity compete with each other, with whatever resources they have, for the differential payoffs that patriarchy allows men.

Men in different societies choose different grounds on which to rank each other. Many societies use the simple facts of age and physical strength to stratify men. The most bizarre and extreme form of patriarchal stratification occurs in those societies which have literally created a class of eunuchs. Our society, reflecting its own particular preoccupations, stratifies men according to physical strength and athletic ability in the early years, but later in life focusses on success with women and ability to make money.

In our society, one of the most critical rankings among men deriving from patriarchal sexual politics is the division between gay and straight men. This division has powerful negative consequences for gay men, and gives straight men privilege. But in addition, this division has a larger symbolic meaning. Our society uses the male heterosexual/homosexual dichotomy as a central symbol for *all* the rankings of masculinity, for the division on *any* grounds between males who are "real men" and have power, and males who are not. Any kind of powerlessness or refusal to compete becomes imbued with the imagery of homosexuality. In the men's movement documentary film *Men's Lives*[3], a high school male who studies modern dance says that others often think he is gay because he is a dancer. When asked why, he gives three reasons: because dancers are "free and loose," because they are "not big like football players," and because "you're not trying to kill anybody." The patriarchal connection: if you are not trying to kill other men, you must be gay.

Another dramatic example of men's use of homosexual derogations as weapons in their power struggle with each other comes from a document that provides one of the richest case studies of the politics of male/male relationships to yet appear: Woodward and Bernstein's *The Final Days* (1976). Ehrlichman jokes that Kissinger is queer, Kissinger calls an un-named colleague a psychopathic homosexual, and Haig jokes that Nixon and Rebozo are having a homosexual relationship. From the highest ranks of male power to the lowest, the gay/straight division is a central symbol of all the forms of ranking and power relations which men put on each other.

The relationships between the patriarchal stratification and competition that men experience with each other and men's patriarchal domination of women are complex. Let us briefly consider several points of interconnection between them. First, women are used as *symbols of success* in men's competition with each other. It is sometimes thought that competition for women is the ultimate source of men's competition with each other. For example, in *Totem and Taboo,* Freud (1960) presented a mythical reconstruction of the origin of society based on sons' sexual competiton with the father, leading to their murdering the father. In this view, if women did not exist, men would not have anything to compete for with each other. There is considerable reason, however, to see women not as the ultimate source of male/male competition, but rather as only symbols in a male contest where real roots lie much deeper.

The recent film, *Paper Chase,* provides an interesting example. This film combines the story of a small group of male law students in their first year of law school with a heterosexual love story between one of the students (played by Timothy Bottoms) and the professor's daughter. As the film develops, it becomes clear that the real business is the struggle within the group of male law students for survival, success, and the professor's blessing—a patriarchal struggle in which several of the less successful are driven out of school and one even attempts suicide. When Timothy

Bottoms gets the professor's daughter at the end, she is simply another one of the rewards he has won by doing better than the other males in her father's class. Indeed, she appears to be a direct part of the patriarchal blessing her father has bestowed on Bottoms.

Second, women often play a mediating role in the patriarchal struggle among men. Women get men together with each other, and provide the social lubrication necessary to smooth over men's inability to relate to each other noncompetitively. This function has been expressed in many myths; for example, the folk tales included in the Grimms' collection about groups of brothers whose younger sister reunites and reconciles them with their king-father, who had previously banished and tried to kill them. A more modern myth, *Deliverance* (Dickey, 1971), portrays what happens when men's relationships with each other are not mediated by women. According to Heilbrun (1972), the central message of *Deliverance* is that when men get beyond the bounds of civilization, which really means beyond the bounds of the civilizing effects of women, men rape and murder each other.

A third function women play in male/male sexual politics is that relationships with women provide men a *refuge* from the dangers and stresses of relating to other males. Traditional relationships with women have provided men a safe place in which they can recuperate from the stresses they have absorbed in their daily struggle with other men, and in which they can express their needs without fearing that these needs will be used against them. If women begin to compete with men and have power in their own right, men are threatened by the loss of this refuge.

Finally, a fourth function of women in males' patriarchal competition with each other is to reduce the stress of competition by serving as an *underclass*. As Janeway (1973; 1975) has written, under patriarchy women represent the lowest status, a status to which men can fall only under the most exceptional circumstances, if at all. Competition among men is serious, but its intensity is mitigated by the fact that there is a lowest possible level to which men cannot fall. One reason men fear women's liberation, writes Janeway, is that the liberation of women will take away this unique underclass status of women. Men will now risk falling lower than ever before, into a new underclass composed of the weak of both sexes. Thus, women's liberation means that the stakes of patriarchal failure for men are higher than they have been before, and that it is even more important for men not to lose.

Thus, men's patriarchal competition with each other makes use of women as symbols of success, as mediators, as refuges, and as an underclass. In each of these roles, women are dominated by men in ways that derive directly from men's struggle with each other. Men need to deal with the sexual politics of their relationships with each other if they are to deal fully with the sexual politics of their relationships with women.

Ultimately, we have to understand that patriarchy has two halves which are intimately related to each other. Patriarchy is a *dual* system, a system in which men oppress women, and in which men oppress themselves and each other. At one level, challenging one part of patriarchy inherently leads to challenging the other. This is one way to interpret why the idea of women's liberation so soon led to the idea of men's liberation, which in my view ultimately means freeing men from the patriarchal sexual dynamics they now experience with each other. But because the patriarchal sexual dynamics of male/male relationships are less obvious than those of male/female relationships, men face a real danger: while the patriarchal oppression of women may be lessened as a result of the women's movement, the patriarchal oppression of men may be untouched. The real danger for men posed by the attack that the women's movement is making on patriarchy is not that this attack will go too far, but that it will not go far enough. Ultimately, men cannot go any further in relating to women as equals than they have been able to go in relating to other men as equals—an equality that has been so deeply disturbing, that has generated so many psychological as well as literal casualties, and has left so many unresolved issues of competition and frustrated love.

MEN'S POWER IN SOCIETY

Let us now consider men's power over women in a third and final context, the context of men's power in the larger society. At one level, men's social identity is defined by the power they have over women, and the power they can compete for against other men. But at another level, most men have very little power over their own lives. How can we understand this paradox?

The major demand to which men must accede in contemporary society is that they play their required role in the economy. But this role is not intrinsically satisfying. The social researcher Yankelovich (1974) has suggested that about 80% of U.S. male workers experience their jobs as intrinsically meaningless and onerous. They experience their jobs and themselves as worthwhile only through priding themselves on the hard work and personal sacrifice they are making to be breadwinners for their families. Accepting these hardships reaffirms their role as family providers and therefore as true men.

Linking the breadwinner role to masculinity in this way has several consequences for men. Men can get psychological payoffs from their jobs that these jobs never provide in themselves. By training men to accept payment for their work in feelings of masculinity rather than in feelings of satisfaction, men will not demand that their jobs be made more meaningful, and as a result jobs can be designed for the more important goal of generating profits. Further, the connection between work and masculinity makes men accept unemployment as their personal failing as males, rather than analyze and change the profit-based economy whose inevitable dislocations make them unemployed or unemployable.

Most critical for our analysis here, men's role in the economy, and the ways men are motivated to play it, has at least two negative effects on women. First, the husband's job makes many direct and indirect demands on wives. In fact, it is often hard to distinguish whether the wife is dominated more by the husband or by the husband's job. The sociologist Turner (1968) writes: "Because the husband must adjust to the demands of his occupation and the family in turn must accommodate to his demands on behalf of his occupational obligations, the husband appears to dominate his wife and children. But as an agent of economic institutions, he perceives himself as controlled rather than as controlling"(p. 282).

Second, linking the breadwinner role to masculinity, in order to motivate men to work, means that women must not be allowed to hold paid work. For the large majority of men who accept dehumanizing jobs only because having a job validates their role as family breadwinner, their wives' taking paid work takes away from them the major and often only way they have of experiencing themselves as having worth. Yankelovich suggests that the frustration and discontent of this group of men whose wives are increasingly joining the paid labor force, is emerging as a major social problem. What these men do to sabotage women's paid work is deplorable, but I believe that it is quite within the bounds of a feminist analysis of contemporary society to see these men as victims as well as victimizers.

One long-range perspective on the historical evolution of the family is that from an earlier stage in which both wife and husband were directly economically productive in the household economic unit, the husband's economic role has evolved so that now it is under the control of forces entirely outside the family. In order to increase productivity, the goal in the design of this new male work role is to increase men's commitment and loyalty to work and to reduce those ties to the family that might compete with it. Men's jobs are increasingly structured as if men had no direct roles or responsibilities in the family—indeed, as if they did not have families at all. But paradoxically, at the same time that men's responsibilities in the family are reduced to facilitate more efficient performance of their work role, the increasing dehumanization of work means that the satisfaction which jobs give men is, to an increasing degree, *only* the satisfaction of fulfilling the family breadwinner role. That is, on the one hand, men's ties to the family have to be broken down to facilitate industrial work discipline, but on the other hand, men's sense of responsibility to the family has to be increased, but shaped into a purely economic form, to provide the motivation for men to work at all. Essential to this process is the transformation of the wife's economic role to providing the supportive services, both physical and psychological, to keep him on the job, and to take over the family responsibilities which his expanded work role will no longer allow him to fulfill himself. The wife is then bound to her husband by her economic dependency on him, and the husband in turn is bound to his job by his family's economic dependence on him.

A final example from the film, *Men's Lives,* illustrates some of these points. In one of the most powerful scenes in the film, a worker in a rubber plant resignedly describes how his bosses are concerned, in his words, with "pacifying" him to get the maximum output from him, not with satisfying his needs. He then takes back this analysis, saying that he is only a worker and therefore cannot really understand what is happening to him. Next, he is asked whether he wants his wife to take a paid job, to reduce the pressure he feels in trying to support his family. In marked contrast to his earlier passive resignation, he proudly asserts that he will never allow her to work, and that in particular he will never scrub the floors after he comes home from his own job. (He correctly perceives that if his wife did take a paid job, he would be under pressure to do some housework.) In this scene, this man expresses and then denies an awareness of his exploitation as a worker. Central to his coping with and repressing his incipient awareness of his exploitation is his false consciousness of his superiority and privilege over women. Not scrubbing floors is a real privilege, and deciding whether or not his wife will have paid work is a real power, but the consciousness of power over his own life that such privilege and power give this man over his life is false. The relative privilege that men get from sexism, and more importantly the false consciousness of privilege men get from sexism, play a critical role in reconciling men to their subordination in the larger political economy. This analysis does not imply that men's sexism will go away if they gain control over their own lives, or that men do not have to deal with their sexism until they gain this control. I disagree with both. Rather my point is that we cannot fully understand men's sexism or men's subordination in the larger society unless we understand how deeply they are related.

To summarize, a feminist understanding of men's power over women, why men have needed it, and what is involved in changing it, is enriched by examining men's power in a broader context. To understand men's power over women, we have to understand the ways in which men feel women have power over them, men's power relationships with other men, and the powerlessness of most men in the larger society. Rectifying men's power relationship with women will inevitably both stimulate and benefit from the rectification of these other power relationships.

REFERENCES

David, D., & Brannon, R. (Eds.). *The forty-nine percent majority: Readings on the male role.* Reading, Mass.: Addison-Wesley, 1975.

Dickey, J. *Deliverance.* New York: Dell, 1971.

Farrell, W. *The liberated man.* New York: Bantam Books, 1975.

Fasteau, M. F. *The male machine.* New York: McGraw-Hill, 1974.

Freud, S. [*Totem and taboo*] (A.A. Brill, trans.). New York: Random, 1960.

Heilbrun, C. G. The masculine wilderness of the American novel. *Saturday Review,* January 29, 1972, 41–44.

Janeway, E. The weak are the second sex. *Atlantic Monthly,* December, 1973, 91–104.

Janeway, E. *Between myth and morning.* Boston: Little, Brown, 1975.

Nichols, J. *Men's liberation: A new definition of masculinity.* Baltimore: Penguin, 1975.

Petras, J. (Ed.). *Sex: Male/gender: Masculine.* Port Washington, New York: Alfred, 1975.

Piercy, M. *Small changes.* New York: Fawcett, 1978.

Pleck, J. H. Men's traditonal attitudes toward women: Conceptual issues in research. In J. Sherman & F. Denmark (Eds.), *The psychology of women: New directions in research.* New York: Psychological Dimensions, in press.

Pleck, J. H., & Sawyer, J. (Eds.). *Men and masculinity.* Englewood Cliffs, N.J.: Prentice-Hall, 1974.

Ryan, W. *Blaming the victim.* New York: Pantheon, 1970.

Turner, R. *Family interaction.* New York: Wiley, 1968.

Woodward, B., & Bernstein, C. *The final days.* Simon & Schuster, 1976.

Yankelovich, D. The meaning of work. In J. Rosow (Ed.), *The worker and the job.* Englewood Cliffs, N.J.: Prentice-Hall, 1974.

FOOTNOTES

[1]See also the *Man's Awareness Network (M.A.N.) Newsletter,* a regularly updated directory of men's movement activities, organizations, and publications, prepared by a rotating group of men's centers (c/o Knoxville Men's Resource Center, PO Box 8060, U.T. Station, Knoxville, Tenn. 37916); and the Men's Studies Collection, Charles Hayden Humanities Library, Massachusetts Institute of Technology, Cambridge, Mass. 02139.

[2]In addition to the mother-domination theory, there are two other psychological theories relating aspects of the early mother/child relationship to men's sexism. The first can be called the "mother identification" theory, which holds that men develop a "feminine" psychological identification because of their early attachment to their mothers, and that men fear this internal feminine part of themselves, seeking to control it by controlling those who actually are feminine—that is, women. The second can be called the "mother socialization" theory, holding that since boys' fathers are relatively absent as sex role models, the major route by which boys learn masculinity is through their mothers' punishing feminine behavior. Thus, males associate women with punishment and pressures to be masculine. Interestingly, these two theories are in direct contradiction, since the former holds that men fear women because women make men feminine, and the latter holds that men fear women because women make men masculine. These theories are discussed at greater length in Pleck (in press).

[3]Available from New Day Films, PO Box 615, Franklin Lakes, NJ 07417.

The Competent Male

JOHN O. CRITES
LOUISE F. FITZGERALD
University of California, Berkeley *(Note 1)

THE CONCEPT OF MALE

The model of the competent male has changed throughout history, with each succeeding age creating and reifying its values through its conception of the image of man. One of the most influential of such models in Western thought was that of the Renaissance man, itself a recreation of the classical Greek ideal. Describing this concept, Kristeller (1972) quotes the Italian philosopher Pico della Mirandelo to explicate the Renaissance notion that man possessed *all* possibilities within himself. Pico's writings presage the modern notion of psychological androgyny (Bem, 1974), implying that Renaissance conceptions of the masculine ideal included the rational faculties, as well as the affective responses labelled more commonly today as feminine. The Renaissance male was truly a *compleat* man, if historians of the period are to be believed (Kristeller, 1972); freed of the rigid constraints of medieval Catholicism, he celebrated the possibility of actualizing all his faculties, a celebration resulting in some of civilization's greatest art, literature, and architecture.

Although historians disagree as to the cultural forces responsible for the fragmentation of the Renaissance ideal, it seems reasonable to trace its roots to the Cartesian world view, the notion of mind/body duality which has profoundly affected modern thought for centuries. The philosophical precursors of this duality can be found in the writings of Reformation theologians, who assigned the rational faculties to males, but warned against the feeling, affective responses (associated with the body) which they relegated to females. This psychological split, originating in a theological ideal of man, was actualized centuries later through the Industrial Revolution which completed the fragmentation by separating man from the home and establishing him once and for all in the rational, instrumental world of work.

Colonial settlers transplanted this European heritage to the New World, where the exigencies of pioneer existence both necessitated and

*Presently at the University of Maryland.

glorified what had by now become the "traditional" masculine qualities. Barker-Benfield (1976) discusses Alexis de Tocqueville's view of the effects of democracy on American men, and on their relations to women. He concludes that the uniquely extreme separation of the sexes in colonial America, based originally on necessity, was glorified through the writings of early authors such as James Fenimore Cooper (*Leatherstocking Tales*) and Ik Marvel (*Reveries of a Bachelor*). The heroes of these works were either lone hunters, or peripatetic bachelors, who personified the masculine ideal of the time: rugged, strong, totally free, totally mobile. D. H. Lawrence describes it starkly, when he writes: "The essential American [male] soul is hard, isolate, stoic and a killer" (Lawrence, 1964). It is in this particular manifestation of the masculine ideal that fear and hatred of women, first found in the writings of Aristotle, became explicit. Marvel remarks that "She will tear the life out of you," a view echoed by a mythical folk hero of the period, Lantern-Jawed Bob, a wandering hunter: "Darn the gals! . . . They're pooty enough to look at, as picters! but to marry one of 'em, an' have her around all the time, huggin' an sich like, would be too much for human nater—turn me into a skeleton if it wouldn't" (Moore, 1963, p. 127). Lantern-Jawed Bob is a philosophical and psychological forebearer of the classical American hero, the western cowboy.

It is only a short way from the frontier tales of Cooper and Marvel to the more contemporary writings of Mailer and Hemingway, Spillane and Fleming. If a culture's values are personified by its literary characters, then the modern masculine ideal appears to be a melange of Stephen Rojack, Mike Hammer, and James Bond—that is, quintessential "macho" male. Such a being is rational, physically impressive, sexually potent, and more than occasionally violent in the attainment of his goals. There appears a total lack of the more tender feelings, and love is unknown—although sexual activity is glorified, often as an act of semiviolence. Although he is intelligent, he is not intellectual—abjuring all cultural pursuits, he appears to satisfy any need for beauty through material acquisition. He has come an exceedingly long way from the Renaissance ideal.

Obviously, the average American male is not a fictional hero: if popular literature embodies our values, it also caricatures them. However, the psychological literature of sex roles clearly demonstrates that the modern male is indeed socialized to value many of the characteristics glorified in adventure and detective stories. The model of the competent male in modern American society includes only instrumental qualities; conspicuous by their absence are such affective traits as gentleness, nurturance, self-disclosure, etc. The masculine ideal not only does not encompass such properties, but actively eschews them as antithetical—with profound consequences for modern man . . . and woman. Split off from half of his nature, man restlessly seeks for it outside of himself. His relationships with women are complicated and often conflicted by the ambivalence of his duality. Longing for what he has been taught to despise, he is often unable to form cooperative, nurturing relationships with either men or women. Becoming a competent male has necessitated living as half a human being.

THE CONTEMPORARY MALE

These historical, literary, and psycho-social images of man across the ages leave his portrait less than complete—indeed, more like that of Dorian Gray, deteriorating in the face of contemporary stresses and strains. And psychology today has little more than general outlines to offer in finishing the picture, but they are a beginning. Pieced together into a more articulate framework they define not only the form but suggest the substance of a coherent conceptualization of the competent male. It centers upon two critical areas of life activity—achievement and affiliation. These are what Freud called *arbeiten und lieben,* work and love (Shoben, 1956), and which, in their fulfillment, he took as the hallmarks of maturity. What problems do they pose for a male in our society, and how does a competent one solve them?

Achievement

Early on in life, the male-child learns that the first arena of achievement and competition is the playground. It is in *play* that the initial conflict with peers occurs for what one wants (Piaget, 1968). The egocentrism of the little boy as he starts school is patent, and it collides headlong with that of other boys (and girls) in the classroom, at recess, and on the way to and from home. Socialized somewhat by its juxtaposition to cooperation, competition for boys nevertheless colors their collective play and constitutes basic training for later achievement in school and sports and in the world-of-work. Through play, they learn what Piaget calls the "rules of the game," conceived not so much to foster cooperation as to control unbridled and unfair competition. What is too frequently grasped, however, is not the rules of the game, but how to get around them—mute testimony to the powerful need to achieve in males even in childhood (McClelland, 1961). A welter of factors contribute to the development of achievement needs, not the least of which are parental injunctions to excel (Steiner, 1974) and mass media glorification of being Number One. A boy grows up thinking that he is less than worthy as a human being if he is not a winner in some activity, particularly sports and preferably contact ones. Achieving in creative pursuits has considerably less valence for boys than girls. Boys soon become aware of a hard-and-fast dictum of sexist socialization: Don't play girls' games, and don't play with girls!

In later *school* and *sports,* the lessons of male childhood come to fruition. The reward system of high school clearly comes down on the side of participation in organized athletics or related "macho" activities. At best, for most adolescent males, school is to be tolerated; at worst, it is a constant source of problems. Statistics indicate that boys are more often disciplined for their classroom behavior, that their academic performance is poorer, and that they more frequently have psychological disorders than their female peers. Of the male youth's dilemma in school, Goldberg (1976, p. 182) observes: "He is taught that 'real boys' are active and strong but then gets into trouble in school for acting like a 'real boy.' " If he conforms to the system by achieving academically, he is rejected in the boy culture as a "sissy." If he chooses to excel in sports, as a way of marking time until graduation, he is even more intensively exposed to sexist socialization. Locker room slogans admonish him to be strong and Spartan: "When the going gets tough, the tough get going"; "Suck up your gut"; "Be No. 1." And national sports figures and folk heroes add: "Winning isn't everything, it's the *only* thing" (Vince Lombardi) and "Losing is like death" (George Allen). No wonder that a mantle of invincibility cloaks a denied vulnerability—but it is nonetheless there. Fear of failure permeates the adolescent life of the young male—in school, in sports, in social relations (Beery, 1975). Particularly is it acute, in an ironically convoluted way, for the scholar athlete who attempts to straddle success in school and sports but is only marginal socially in both areas. So much for the Renaissance man in contemporary school society.

Similarly, in the realm of *work* the adult male must put on a "straightjacket of success" in order to achieve. A recent editorial in a man's magazine enumerates what capacities are necessary for surviving in the modern corporation, including: "be able to obey rules and follow orders, regardless of how silly and unnecessary they may seem"; "ability to control and hide true feelings when faced with an incompetent superior"; "can be intensely loyal to an employer, yet able to transfer that loyalty when you change jobs." What manner of man do these prescriptions for success portray? One who is expedient, shallow, conforming but competitive, and ultimately ruthless. And one who is willing to subject himself to humiliation—what Goldberg (1976) refers to as "brutalization" and the magazine article terms "hazing"; "Bosses tease and put down inferiors to assert their authority, and many employees wind up feeling humiliated." All this to further what Horney (1950) calls the "Search for Glory"—an all-consuming drive for perfection, success, and vindictive triumph. Goaded on to greater effort by his Pig Parent (Steiner, 1974; Horney's "Tyranny of the Should"), the striving male falls victim to the process he presumably controls, and he loses power over his life. As Sherwood Anderson asked of another generation, not unlike ours in their pursuit of materialistic success: "What price glory?" For the contemporary male, the price is great, both physically and psychically: higher mortality, more suicides, greater incidence of fatal diseases (cardiovascular, cirrhosis of the liver, pneumonia, tuberculosis, etc.), more migraines, ulcers, hypertension, alcoholism, less tolerance for stress, and more pervasive interpersonal isolation than women (Goldberl, 1976, Ch. 12). Achievement for the contemporary male leaves much to be desired.

Affiliation

Man fares even less well in his attempts at affiliation. Again, basic training takes place in childhood, the salient variables being the *parental attitudes* boys are reared under in the home. Roe (1957), Bayley and Schaefer (1960), Symonds (1939) have identified three interpersonal orientations which predominate in the family: acceptance, avoidance, and concentration. Of these it is the latter two which have the greatest salience for the development of the contemporary male. The psychological mien of the father is an attitude of avoidance, of calculated aloofness and distance which conveys the "strong and silent" (undemonstrative and noncommunicative) values of the man to the boy. The main attitude of the mother is that of concentration, which at once fosters the boy's dependence upon women for emotional nurturance yet enjoins them to be nurturing and life-supporting when they grow up. Because of the one-sided injunctions of the father and the mixed messages of the mother, boys are scripted to be half-men, as shown in Figure 1. In this transactional structural analysis of the adult male (Steiner, 1974, p. 168), his characteristic modes of affiliating are thrown into bold relief: his strong Adult keeps him rational and logical, "straight thinking"; his weak nurturing Parent precludes contradictory "soft" feelings of compassion, empathy, understanding, etc.; his strong Pig Parent (the mother's Parent in his Child) tells him what he *should* do to be a "real man," "to be out of touch with [his] nurturing, intuitive, or fun-loving feelings" (Steiner, 1974, p. 167); and, his weak Little Professor and Natural Child complement the strictures of the strong Pig Parent.

These ego states carry over directly to his *relationships with other men,* who have largely been scripted the same way. When men meet, the result is essentially a "noninteraction," either a glad-handing, back-slapping superficiality or a self-conscious interchange of monosyllables, caricatured by Gary Cooper's taciturn cowboy who says little more than "Yep." Goldberg (1976), p. 137 observes that:

"From both ends of the continuum, men seem to be blocked when they try to relate to each other. That is, they are not comfortable sharing their down sides—their failures, anxieties, and disappointments. Perhaps they fear being seen as weak, complaining losers or crybabies, a perception that threatens their masculine images. Neither do they seem to feel comfortable sharing their ecstasies or successes for fear of inciting competitive jealousies or appearing boastful. Consequently, verbal social interactions between men focus on neutral, largely impersonal subject matters such as automobiles, sports, and politics." Inhibited in moving towards other men on any deeper emotional level by strong internalized taboos and constrained in moving against them by externally imposed sanctions, the

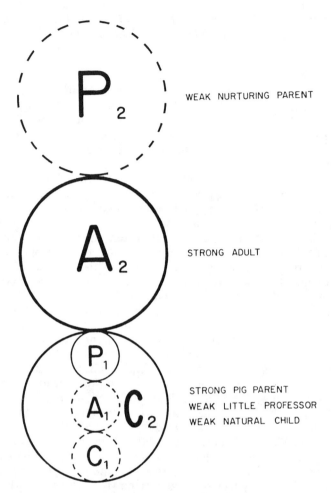

WEAK NURTURING PARENT

STRONG ADULT

STRONG PIG PARENT
WEAK LITTLE PROFESSOR
WEAK NATURAL CHILD

Figure 1. Male sex role scripting. From *Scripts People Live,* by C. Steiner. Copyright 1974 by Claude Steiner. Reprinted by permission of Grove Press, Inc.

contemporary male has only the way out—to move away (Horney, 1946, 1950). At first, it is only a moving away from others; ultimately, it can be a more radical moving away from self, and alienation and externalization which is the epitome of interpersonal isolation.

In his *relationships with women,* the contemporary male experiences even greater problems in fulfilling his affiliation needs than in relating to men. Too often he narrowly defines these relationships as sexual ones only. Or, at the other extreme, he idealizes women much as he may have his mother. Goldberg (1976, p. 31) describes man's search for an "earth mother," "women willing to play the role of the old-fashioned, selfless, passive, and devoted female," who complements the incomplete male, as depicted in Figure 2A (Steiner, 1974, p. 174). Here can be seen graphically the pitiful attempt of two half-people to become a whole. In the male, the Adult ego state is strongest and usually "takes charge" in the world for the female, whose Adult is weak. Conversely, the female's strong Parent nurtures the male's Child ("little boy") in the home. If they marry and "become one" (Figure 2B), the composite they create is neither a fully functioning man nor woman. And in this misbegotten psyche are the seeds of its own destruction: two Pig Parents (P_1) in constant contention if not open combat. If they separate, man is again left with a weak nurturing Parent, but he is older, more isolated, more susceptible to mental illness, and more likely to commit suicide than before (Goldberg, 1976).

The Modal Contemporary Male

Not all men, of course, fit the modal personality pattern of the contemporary male, but enough do that it has cogency for most. From boyhood through manhood, sexist socialization transmits and rewards certain stereotyped behaviors and values for men which are highly valued in our society. The ideal man "stands alone": he is independent, strong, logical, fearless, controlled, and unemotional. He is stalwart and steadfast under stress, imaginative and ingenious when solving problems, and dedicated and persevering in accomplishing tasks. He is expected to deal successfully with the "outer world" and not have to cope with the "inner world." But his feelings and emotions are every bit as real as his more objective experiences. They impinge upon him in his work, where the single most important factor in job failure is inability to "get along with others" (Crites, 1969), and they intrude upon his interpersonal life, where he finds he has fewer meaningful relationships with both men and women. It is ironical though hardly surprising, then, that at his presumed pinnacle of power in mid-life the contemporary male may face critical crises of existential proportions. What is he to do? Perls (1969, p. 40) answers: "It's the awareness, the full experience . . . of how you are stuck, that makes you recover, and realize the whole thing is just a nightmare. . . ."

THE COMPETENT MALE

If the contemporary male is to become the competent male, he must redefine what he means by achievement and success. Too long has he judged himself by external standards of competition, always relative to the accomplishments of others. A change of frame is needed (Watzlawick, Weakland, & Fisch, 1974), a shift in locus from the external to the internal

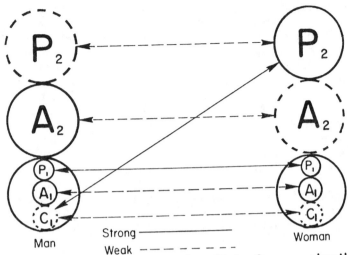

A. A woman and a man: Sex-Role Communication

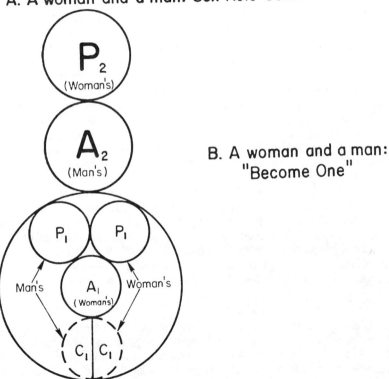

B. A woman and a man: "Become One"

Figure 2. Traditional sex roles for a woman and a man. From *Scripts People Live*, by C. Steiner. Copyright 1974 by Claude Steiner. Reprinted by permission of Grove Press, Inc.

in order to capture the essence of *competence* (White, 1959). To be competent is to experience mastery of self and fulfillment of potentialities. Super (1951, p. 7) eloquently defines it this way:

" 'Success,' as the world judges it, is fruitless and empty unless it is also seen as success by the individual. What would wealth have been to Ghandi, or the love and respect of humble men and women to Bismarck? What use had Thoreau for prestige and status, or Theodore Roosevelt for opportunities to be alone with himself and the universe? In the eyes of each of these persons, and of some others, each of them was a failure. Individual values and hence individual judgments, differ in such matters." Each man can define his own criterion of excellence and take pride in the progressive approximation of it, without reference to others. If internal standards conducive to personal growth and development are met, then external competition is meaningless, because it is subsumed by what a man already is. Rather than being continually caught up in a maelstrom of competition, he can be free to cooperate with others toward the attainment of common goals.

Likewise, in interpersonal relationships he can be free to enjoy equality if he supplants competition with cooperation. He can wean himself from his emotional dependency upon women by relinquishing his assumed superiority and relating to them as equals. Steiner (1974, p. 239) diagrams liberated communication between a woman and man in Figure 3. As contrasted with traditional transactions (Figure 2A), these emanate from fully developed ego states. The man's nurturing Parent has become stronger as have his intuitive Little Professor (A_1) and his funloving, sexy Natural Child (C_1); conversely, the woman's Adult has grown more powerful and her Natural Child has opened up. The Pig Parents of both have been "decommissioned," and are not allowed to exert an influence upon the rest of the personality. The ensuing relationship is a cooperative one free of inequalities, power-plays, and rescues. It is a relationship in which a man can be independent as well as interdependent with a woman. And, it is much the same kind of relationship he can establish with other men. No longer need he relate to them on only an Adult or Pig Parent level; he can get in touch with their feelings as well as his own through his Little Professor and he can offer solace and strokes with his Nurturing Parent. Slowly but surely a network of "buddyships," as Goldberg (1976) calls them, comes into being, and, along with his newly framed relationships with women, the competent male finds that he has a satisfying and supportive system of affiliation with others where once he stood in isolation.

If the cardinal trait of the contemporary male is competition, then that of the modal competent male is cooperation. Horney (1946, 1950) might well have included still another mode in her system of interpersonal orientations: moving *with* people. For this way of relating to others, both on the job and off, commends itself personally as well as socially. Recently completed research at the Institute of Human Development, University of California (Berkeley), indicated that a social *maturity* factor for males in a longitudinal study, defined by high Dominance, Socialization, Responsibility, and Tolerance with low Good Impression and Communality on the California Psychological Inventory, was correlated with several criteria of

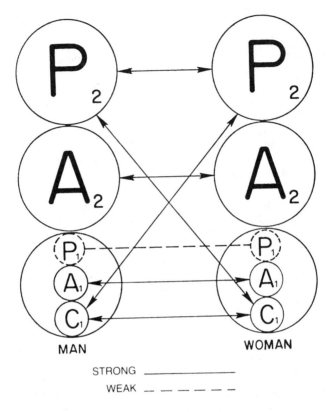

Figure 3. Liberated communication between a man and a woman. From *Scripts People Live,* by C. Steiner. Copyright 1974 by Claude Steiner. Reprinted by permission of Grove Press, Inc.

integrative adjustment, such as better overall health, fewer drinking problems, and more satisfying interpersonal relationship (Brooks, Note 2). This empirical description of the competent male is consonant with a concept of androgyny appropriate to both men and women, as summarized by Fasteau (1975, p. 196):

"Perhaps in the future, our lives will be shaped by a view of personality which will not assign fixed ways of behaving to individuals on the basis of sex. Instead, it would acknowledge that each person has the potential to be—depending on the circumstances—both assertive *and* yielding, independent *and* dependent, job- *and* people-oriented, strong *and* gentle, in short, both 'masculine' *and* 'feminine'; that the most effective and happy individuals are likely to be those who have accepted and developed both these 'sides' of themselves; and that to deny either is to mutilate and deform; that human beings, in other words, are naturally androgynous."

REFERENCE NOTES

1. Both a man and a woman have collaborated on this paper because neither can know the other alone.
2. Brooks, J. B. *Social maturity and its developmental antecedents.* Unpublished manuscript, Institute of Human Development, University of California (Berkeley), 1978.

REFERENCES

Bayley, N., & Schaefer, E. S. Relationships between socioeconomic variables and the behavior of mothers toward young children. *Journal of Genetic Psychology,* 1960, *96*, 61–77.

Barker-Benfield, G. J. *The horrors of the half-known life.* New York: Harper & Row, 1976.

Beery, R. G. Fear of failure in the student experience. *Personnel and Guidance Journal,* 1975, *54*, 191–203.

Bem, S. L. The measurement of psychological androgyny. *Journal of Consulting and Clinical Psychology,* 1974, *42*, 155–162.

Crites, J. O. *Vocational psychology.* New York: McGraw-Hill, 1969.

Fasteau, M. F. *The male machine.* New York: Dell, 1975.

Goldberg, H. *The hazards of being male.* New York: Nash, 1976.

Horney, K. *Our inner conflicts.* New York: Norton, 1946.

Horney, K. *Neurosis and human growth.* New York: Norton, 1950.

Kristeller, P. O. *Renaissance concepts of man.* New York: Harper & Row, 1972.

Lawrence, D. H. *Studies in classic American literature.* New York: Viking, 1964.

McClelland, D. C. *The achieving society.* Princeton: Van Nostrand, 1961.

Moore, A. *The frontier mind.* New York: McGraw-Hill, 1963.

Perls, F. S. *Gestalt therapy verbatim.* Lafayette, Calif.: Real People Press, 1969.

Piaget, J. *Six psychological studies.* New York: Vintage, 1968.

Roe, A. Early determinants of vocational choice. *Journal of Counseling Psychology,* 1957, *4*, 212–217.

Shoben, E. J., Jr. Work, love, and maturity. *Personnel and Guidance Journal,* 1956, *34*, 326–332.

Steiner, C. *Scripts people live.* New York: Grove, 1974.

Super, D. E. Vocational adjustment: Implementing a self-concept. *Occupations,* 1951, *30*, 88–92.

Symonds, P. M. *The psychology of parent-child relationships.* New York: Appleton-Century-Crofts, 1939.

Watzlawick, J. H., Weakland, J. H., & Fisch, R. *Change: Principles of problem formation and problem resolution.* New York: Norton, 1974.

White, R. W. Motivation reconsidered: The concept of competence. *Psychological Review,* 1959, *66*, 297–333.

The Male Role and Heterosexual Behavior

ALAN E. GROSS

University of Missouri, St. Louis*

The intent of this paper is to extract those elements of the traditional male sex role which have relevance for sexual behavior and to suggest how they influence adult male heterosexual behavior in contemporary Western society. Two important themes—the centrality of sexual behavior to male gender identity, and the relative isolation of sex from other aspects of male heterosocial relationships—are identified. Then a number of linkages between male sexual behaviors/attitudes and general facets of the male sex role are examined: (a) goals and success, (b) control and power, and (c) aggression and violence. It is argued that many of the influences emanating from a restrictive sex-typed socialization process are maladaptive, and specifically that recent shifts away from the traditional "sexual animal" stereotype toward a modern "competent lover" image are largely surface alterations, that both have their roots in the same learning process with similar pernicious effects.

The viewpoint of this paper, following Gagnon and Simon (1973), is that human sexual behavior just as most other social behavior is largely acquired through experience and socialization. Further, the different socialization experiences of men and women are major contributors to their respective sexual attitudes and behaviors. In keeping with the theme of this journal issue, my intent here is to extract those elements of the traditional male sex role which have relevance for sexual behavior, and to suggest how they influence adult male heterosexual behavior in contemporary Western society.

I am grateful to Joseph Pleck for insightful and supportive suggestions; to Pleck, Clyde Hendrick, and Elaine Walster for providing bibiliographic materials; and to Annie Q. Fitzgerald and Nancy Felipe Russo for helpful comments.

*Now at the University of Maryland.

"Male sex role" is neither a unitary nor an unchanging concept. Especially in a time of dynamic change, it is difficult to identify the complex and sometimes contradictory set of behaviors that comprise the male role and the subset that define the male sexual role. But even lacking a precise and exhaustive definition, it is possible to identify some general sexual themes and to explore the socialization processes which underlie them. A number of agreed-upon qualities have been identified as typically more male than female (Bem, 1974; Broverman, Broverman, Clarkson, Rosenkrantz, & Vogel, 1972). Recently several writers have attempted to codify these qualities into suggested male themes or types. For example, Sawyer (1970) has suggested the stereotypic man is a dominator-achiever and a closed individual who finds it difficult to express emotion. And Brannon (1976) has emphasized four pervasive imperatives which boys learn to identify with maleness as they grow up: avoid typical female behavior, achieve success, don't be dependent on anyone else, and be aggressive. These and other attempts to define the male sex role contain a number of concepts and associated behaviors which have implications for heterosexual relationships.

To begin this analysis, I will discuss how two distinctly male sexual themes—the central importance of sexual behavior to male gender identity and the relative isolation of sex from other aspects of male heterosocial relationships—emerge from learning experiences. Then a number of linkages between male sexual behaviors/attitudes and general facets of the male sex role will be examined: (a) goals and success, (b) control and power, and (c) aggression and violence. Finally, it will be suggested that recent changes away from a traditional "sexual animal" stereotype toward a modern "competent lover" image are largely surface alterations, that both traditional and modern male heterosexual patterns are shaped by the same basic male ethos.

TWO MALE SEXUAL THEMES

Sex is perceived as more important and enjoyable for men than for women. Reik has observed that "sometimes men feel that they have to have sexual intercourse for hygenic reasons, just as they have to eat three meals daily" (1960, p. 128).[1] The implication of Reik's comment and many others like it is that sex is important, central, and even necessary for men. This kind of statement is often based on assumptions that male sexuality is more biologically than experientially determined, and that biological sexual effects are stronger in men than women (Bardwick, 1970, 1971; Kaats & Davis, 1972). Explanations such as Bardwick's, which tightly link sex to biology, have not gone unchallenged. Although feminists and others who

[1]This and all other quotations from this source are excerpts from *Sex In Man and Woman*, by Theodor Reik. Copyright © 1960 by Theodor Reik. Reprinted by permission of Farrar, Straus & Giroux, Inc.

attempt to create increased awareness of restrictive sex-role behaviors have successfully debunked some of the more blatant physiological sexual fictions—for example, masturbation-caused insanity, vaginal orgasm (Koedt, 1970; Masters & Johnson, 1966), the belief that men have stronger sex drives than women persists, with no compelling evidence to support it. (Byrne, 1977).

Whether myth or biological fact, men and women generally believe and act as if sex is more central, enjoyable, and necessary for males. For example, responses to an extensive series of interviews with married couples (Rainwater, 1965) indicate that husbands, especially those in the lower economic classes, are much more likely than their wives to find sex enjoyable. A typical husband in Rainwater's sample asserts, "Sex is the most important thing, say 95% of marriage" (p. 83). In contrast, many wives in the same sample simply tolerate sex: "He thinks sex is very important. . . . He couldn't live without it, I guess. . . . Me, I could do without it; our feelings are completely opposite" (p. 113). Additional evidence that sex is perceived as more important for men than for women is reported by Peplau, Rubin, and Hill (1977). In their questionnaire study of college dating couples, males rated "desire for sexual activity" as a more important dating goal than did their female partners. And in a very recent study (Crain & Roth, Note 1), both husbands and wives living in university married student housing attributed husbands' sexual initiations more to "inner need."

Some men have escaped or resisted socialization forces which encourage them to sexualize relationships, but even these men are usually aware that they must meet the general sexual expectations of others to be considered truly manly. A particularly poignant example of a boy attempting to fulfill sexual role expectations was related in a letter to Ann Landers (1976). The 16-year-old letter writer, responding to a previous letter in which a 15-year-old girl lamented that she had to either "put out or sit home," revealed why the boys in his crowd were sexually aggressive with girls: "Most of us try because we think it's expected. But it's a relief when the answer is no. Then we don't have to prove anything."

The central importance of sexuality in masculine identity probably begins early in boyhood and can be explained by a combination of social and biological forces. Boys begin masturbating earlier than girls (Kinsey, Pomeroy, & Martin, 1948); they typically learn about masturbation from other boys (Gagnon & Henderson, 1975). It is likely that boys begin masturbating earlier than girls because their external genitalia are more accessible to manipulation and because erections call attention to the penis. Gagnon and Simon comment: "masturbation tends to focus the male sense of feeling or sexual desire in the penis, giving the genitals centrality" (1973, p. 62). Heterosexual problems associated with genital/sexual focusing are closely related to and compounded by a tendency in men to isolate sexual activity from other significant facets of social life.

Men tend to isolate sex from other social aspects of life. A major consequence of early genital focus, reinforced in adolescence by heavy peer pressure to seek sex in order to validate masculinity (Kanin, 1967), is that men tend to experience sex as separate from other social and psychological aspects of living. At the extreme this tendency may manifest itself as an overwhelming or even exclusive emphasis on sexuality in a relationship. It is probably true that in recent years the purely sexual male image has assumed more subtle forms, but these new low-key seduction styles seem more surface adaptations than evidence that men have relinquished the basic belief that it is necessary to be "on the make" to be masculine. Even Woody Allen in *Play It Again Sam* recognizes that male fulfillment comes from sexual conquest; the comedy results from his fumbling and bizarre attempts to mimic a "real man" (Bogart) in wooing the female sexual object.

In addition to early genital focus and peer pressure to sexually validate masculinity, several additional explanations have been offered for the male propensity to separate sex from love and affection. Fasteau (1974) hypothesizes that isolated sex is a defense against male vulnerability. He believes that when men allow themselves to combine sexual attraction and intimacy, they become dependent on their partner, and that this kind of dependency, especially on a woman, is not compatible with the internalized masculine idea. A more general explanation for the reluctance of some males to establish deep intimate bonds with women is that women are generally viewed unfavorably (Broverman et al., 1972; McKee & Sherriffs, 1957), and that men, especially men concerned about their masculinity, feel hesitant to relate closely to women because the association is potentially stigmatizing (Brannon, 1976).

Certainly a picture of the male as interested only in isolated sex is overdrawn but there are recent data which indicate that men more than women are likely to view any heterosexual relationship in a sexual-romance framework (Rytting, 1975). College males in Rytting's study less often made distinctions between friendly and sexual relationships, and were more likely to expect sex as part of the relationship. Additional support for the view of men as evaluating heterosexual relationships along a central sexual-romantic dimension comes from Guinsburg's (1973) study of platonic and romantic relationships. Males in this study had difficulty distinguishing the two kinds of relationships. Rytting (Note 2) interprets these two studies as yielding a "picture of the undifferentiating male making quantitative distinctions along a single continuum of romantic-sexual involvement relatively divorced from emotional and intellectual involvement . . . in contrast with the discriminating woman seeing sexual and emotional involvement as integrated in a romantic relationship." From the sex differences which emerge in his study, Rytting proposes that definitions of intimacy from masculine and feminine perspectives differ: Men view "sex as being ubiquitous and therefore a focal point for all relationships with woman," while women distinguish sexual from nonsexual intimacy. Drawing on additional data, especially a negative correlation between perceived sexual behavior and verbal intimacy for the males, Rytting concludes that the male perspective leads to indiscriminate sexual decision making and, even worse, tends to inhibit intimacy.

Theodor Reik (1960) not only agrees that males typically fixate on sex in relations with females, but he also suggests that the male sexual orientation is incompatible with the more extensive social and affectional needs of many women. Reik contends that those who analyze heterosexual relations often fail to distinguish needs for affection *(besoin de tendresse)* from sexual desire *(besoin de volupte),* and to recognize that the first is stronger in women and the second stronger in men. He notes that "after sexual intercourse women often feel the wish that their partner should express his love . . . such a need is very rarely experienced by the man after sexual intercourse. It is as though for him all was said and done in the sexual act" (p. 127).

Sexual problems between men and women often develop because genital focus and subsequent sexual isolation in the male is out of phase with female development. Gagnon and Henderson (1975) have outlined some of the problems that emerge when boys and girls first meet each other sexually in adolescence:

> The young male, pressed on by his male peers and his prior masculinity training . . . pushes for more sexual activity when dating. Conversely, many young females . . . spend a good deal of time preventing sexual intimacy. Therefore, because of earlier differences in learning how to be sexual, males committed to sexuality but less trained in affection and love, may interact with females who are committed to love but relatively untrained in sexuality [p. 38].

These difficulties are not limited to youth. Many adult men find it difficult or impossible to integrate heterosexual sex with friendship. In the worst cases, sex becomes so incompatible with emotional closeness that it actually seems to preempt intimacy. Lillian Rubin (1976), who conducted extensive interviews with 75 working class and professional married couples, summarizes the incompatible consequences of male and female socialization:

> Man's everpresent sexual readiness is not simply an expression of urgent sexual need but also a complex compensatory response to a socialization process that *constricts* the development of the emotional side of his personality in all but sexual expression . . . [but for the woman there is a process] that encourages the development of the emotional side of her personality in all but sexual expression [p. 50].

It is not surprising that Freud (1905/1963) recognized the general problem of fusing sex and affection: "To ensure a fully normal attitude in love, two currents of feeling have to unite . . . the tender affectionate feelings and the sensual feelings'' (p. 1).[2]

Thus sex and social pressures about sex become important early in boyhood and are maintained as an important element in masculine identity throughout much of adult life. Compared to women, men tend not only to focus more on sexuality with cross-sex partners, but also to isolate sex from other aspects of heterosexual relating. This sex difference is both reflected and maintained by numerous features of Western culture. Purely pornographic materials as well as slick sexually-oriented magazines of the *Playboy* genre are aimed at the male market, while emotional love stories are typically found in women's publications. Even the language used by boys and men to denote sexual intercourse is more explicitly sexual and frequently aggressive—for example, ''screw,'' ''fuck,'' ''bang''—as contrasted with favored female phrases for coitus, such as ''make love with,'' ''go to bed with,'' which extend the context and diminish sexual/genital connotations (Sanders, Note 3).

Whatever the evolution of the tendency for men to separate sex from other social interaction, it is clear that the effects of this separation are usually destructive. Traditional male socialization has prevented many men from experiencing potentially rich heterosexual relationships which combine sex and affection, and it has restricted men from forming close platonic relationships with half of humanity. Unfortunately the divorce of sex from affection is not the only negative legacy of the male socialization process.

GOALS AND SUCCESS

One of the dominant themes that a boy learns as he approaches manhood is that success in his work is important, and that success is operationalized in terms of specific goals. The American male has been characterized as having his eye so firmly fixed on objectives as he attempts to climb the status ladder that he is unconcerned with the present quality of his life. This achievement theme has some obvious implications when it is transferred from the work place to the sexual arena.

The most direct parallel to goal orientation at work is orgasm orientation in bed. Preoccupation with orgasm as an indicator of sexual accomplishment not only applies to the traditional male's selfish attempts to satisfy himself, but it extends to the modern male-lover's preoccupation with bringing his partner to climax. As Fasteau (1974) puts it, ''Since orgasm is thought to be the only real point of making love, physically competent performance, delivering the goods, easily becomes the sole basis for men's sexual self-esteem'' (p. 27).

---

[2] A study by Tharp (1963) provides an exception to the male pattern of separation of sex from affection; it indicates that sex and intimacy can be related, at least for some monogamous, educated men in their mid-forties. Sheehy (1976) provides some anecdotal support for this possibility.

The development of goal/orgasm orientation may be related to early sexual experience. As noted, boys are commonly introduced to sex via masturbation (Kinsey et al., 1948), and teenage masturbation, especially when it is socially compared and discussed among peers, typically focuses on orgasm. Boys who (claim they) can ejaculate fastest, farthest, and most often, either privately or in such games as "circle-jerk," receive social praise and reinforcement. Teen peer groups do not, to my knowledge, award prizes for the best feeling or most thrilling masturbatory experience. Unfortunately, this kind of socialization augurs poorly for later heterosexual adjustment. As boys shift from auto-erotic to social sex, it is likely that they will persist in evaluating sexual success against quantitative criteria. It is not surprising that traditional adult men still count mental notches for each sexual partner or even for each sexual act, while more sophisticated modern men count the number of orgasms they "produce" for their partners. And in some subcultures, this quantitative approach to sexuality expresses itself as a positive association between degree of masculinity and number of children.

Sometimes such sexual goal orientation causes problems for men. Julty (1972), in discussing causes of impotence, clearly points a blaming finger at the male success script: "But it's that damned goal orientation which messes us up and takes its toll . . . the dates, talks, exchanges of feelings . . . are not stations of enjoyment . . . they are only fueling stops . . . Orgasm doth not a relationship make."

While the orgasm itself is a specific goal, many men consider the entire sexual encounter as a goal. Fasteau (1974) observes that "For most men, courting and seduction are nuisances. The focus is almost exclusively on reaching the goal of conquest with all possible speed" (p. 32). Whether the goal is general—"conquest"—or more specific—orgasm—men's concerns with ends often cheat them of process pleasures. Moreover, some women have become aware of how they have been cheated by men's aim orientation. Bengis (1972), having turned to a woman for the sexual intimacy she has missed with men, provides a relevant comparison: "For men sex was aim oriented. There was a beginning, a middle, and an end . . . (with a woman) the real pleasure came from intimacy in all its forms . . . There was just being close" (p. 161).

When sex is perceived as goal rather than process, a man may come to value sexual activities not according to his own feelings, but contingent on the feedback he receives from his partner. And women, not insensitive to the frailty of the male sexual ego, often collude by providing the positive responses the man seems to need, ranging from mild verbal praise to passionate histrionics; in one survey (Tavris, 1973) more than two-thirds of women reported faking orgasm.

It is not uncommon for men to seek rewards that lie outside of the relationship itself. Early in adolescence, most boys recognize that sexual success is not "scoring" in the parked car, but describing real or imagined sexual exploits to a group of teen-age cronies the next day at school or even the same night at the local drive-in. Thus, the sexual partner becomes a mere instrumentality used by boys to achieve status in the eyes of those who really count, the male peer group. Kanin (1967) reports that more than 65% of his undergraduate male interviewees indicated that their friends had exerted pressure on each other "to seek premarital sex experience" (p. 497). And looking outside of the sexual relationship for personal payoff doesn't end in adolescence. For example, Korda (1973) explains the complex posturing and Goffmanesque face-work by which men attempt to communicate their sexual prowess and success to fellow males at the office: "An office affair is a badge of status, always provided that it's handled well."

Perhaps the most deleterious consequence of the male obsession with goals and success is that honest communication is often inhibited between men and their sexual partners. Success or the appearance of success becomes so important to the man that he cannot—and his partner knows he cannot—tolerate critical comments or even friendly suggestions related to his sexual functioning. Even when women are not used as a means of gaining acceptance with a male peer group, men are often more concerned with preserving their image as "real men" than with open and constructive interchange. The various defensive arrangements that men have constructed with sexual partners may serve well to reduce threat of failure and to save face, but in many cases this protection is bought at the expense of a more complete, human, and mutually enjoyable sexual experience.

CONTROL AND POWER

Solely by virtue of their sex, many men are officially recognized by the U.S. Bureau of the Census as "head of household." This formal label is probably an accurate reflection of the powerful family position occupied by Western males. Even (or especially) when males are frustrated in their attempts to gain power at work or in other settings that they can't control, they have learned to expect, establish, and maintain control at home and in social relationships.

Not surprisingly, characteristic male behaviors and attitudes associated with maintaining control and power at work and home are commonly found in sexual relationships as well. One means by which a man maintains sexual control is to play the role of initiator. Carlson (1976) analyzed responses from a sample of husbands and wives in an attempt to discover if the traditional male sexual-initiator norm still holds. Of the husbands, 44% felt that husbands should assume the chief responsibility for making sexual overtures, but 45% felt that the responsibility for sexual initiation should be equal. About half of the wives in Carlson's sample agreed that the husband should be the initiator, 26% thought the responsibility should be shared, and the remainder refused to assign the responsibility to either spouse. As encouraging as these data may appear to those who favor sexual egalitarianism, it should be noted that virtually no one indicated that the wife should be the primary initiator, and that a substantial group still favored the traditional husband's role. Interestingly, the belief that men should make the initial sexual advances was expressed more often by upper-middle-class husbands. Carlson concludes that the "initiation of sexual activity is (still) viewed by both spouses as being a husband-oriented activity" (p.105). A very recent study of college-educated young marrieds yielded data which corroborate Carlson's results that husbands are the primary initiators (Crain and Roth, Note 1). And Peplau et al. (1977) note that virtually all of the men in their sample of college couples exert positive control by playing the role of initiator.

Of course the societal prescription for male initiation and against female sexual assertiveness is not limited to marriage, where there are perhaps less sanctions against women acting as initiators. The widespread norm against female sexual initiation is brutally illustrated in the classic 1953 film, *The Wild Ones*. Johnny (played by Marlon Brando), a tough motorcycle gang leader, having just rescued Kathy, a local waitress, from a group of rival bikers, finds himself alone with her in a quiet wooded area. Kathy attempts to put her arms tenderly around Johnny, but Johnny responds by savagely kissing her and barking, "Right now I can knock you around . . . I don't even want to know you." Although Johnny's reaction reflects part of a complex male script involving aggression and the separation of sex from affection, his rejection of Kathy probably stems in part from her violation of the initiation norm and his need to reassert male control.

The initiation norm that prescribes that the man must make the first sexual move is usually extended to prescribe male control during the sexual interaction itself. Although men, by mutual consent of both sexual partners, usually choreograph and direct the sex act, some recent results from a national probability sample (Hunt, 1976) indicate that only 22% of men admit disliking having a female take the sexual lead. It is possible that Hunt's respondents were attempting to present themselves in a socially desirable manner as modern egalitarians; moreover there are no known data indicating that women dislike having men take the lead, probably because the question has not been asked.

Safilios-Rothschild (1977) believes that even contemporary women feel uncomfortable taking the sexual lead and that their discomfort may be related to their empathy with the male's fear of losing control: "[Men are] ambivalent in their reactions toward sexually active and skilled women" (p. 112). And some of Komarovsky's (1976) intensive interviews with college males support the notion that men have difficulty accepting sexual invitations from women. For example, after expounding about how he wanted "a girl to be sexually liberated, to be ready to sleep with me, perhaps even on the first or second night," one of Komarovsky's liberal informants describes a situation in which a "beautiful, 21-year-old co-ed" suggested a sexual encounter with him after which he "didn't feel too good about it and I'll not see her again . . . maybe I was taken aback by her forwardness" (p. 91).

One of the most limiting features of the controlling male sex role, especially in sexual relationships, is the requirement that men are not allowed to reveal ignorance or even uncertainty. The combination of the male posing as expert or teacher and the female deferring to "superior" male knowledge often inhibits couples from being open to improving their sexual interaction. Masters and Johnson (1970) point out: "The assumption . . . by both men and women, that sexual expertise is the man's responsibility constantly interferes with effective sexual functioning" (p. 87).

The male role of sexual expert is closely related to a general male caveat against help-seeking. Rugged independence even when inappropriate or harmful, has become an integral part of traditional masculinity. This is illustrated in a modern fable dealing with the socialization of a young boy (Allen, 1972). The boy is instructed: "You must never ask anyone for help, or even let anyone know that you are confused or frightened. That's part of learning to be a man." In sexual matters, so central to the male ego, admitting ignorance, asking for information, or seeking help are especially difficult. In a recent survey, Skovholt, Nagy, and Epting (Note 4) found that college men were significantly less able than college women to ask sexual questions of a friend.

Because men are assumed (even by themselves) to be sexually knowledgeable, sexual information sometimes is acquired only accidentally and, unfortunately for men and their partners, relatively late in life. For example, Singer (1976), in a not atypical autobiographical account of male sex life, describes how in his late twenties, after experiencing a variety of sexual relationships, he "listened to a [radio] conversation . . . about the difference between clitoral and vaginal orgasms [and realized that I] didn't know what a clitoris was." Such lack of basic sexual information is not uncommon even among relatively educated men, and of course the state of ignorance is maintained by the complicity of female partners who are fearful, often with justification, of injuring the male ego and/or damaging the relationship.

The hypothesis that men are hesitant to publicly seek out sexual information is corroborated by Nichols (1975) who reports that a midwestern university class titled Problems in Human Sexuality drew 40 students, the large majority of them women. Although the relative absence of men evidently puzzled some observers, a female sociology professor offered a succinct explanation: "Most males are pigheaded and think they know all there is to know about sex" (p. 198). Nichols concludes that "men pretend to know because such knowledge is part of the facade required by masculinist values. . . . To be 'in control' one must 'know' and hence a know-it-all pose is used as a means of convincing others that one is masterfully erotic" (p.199).

This male attitude toward admitting ignorance publicly may explain the tremendous burgeoning of sex manuals in the past few years. Although some of these manuals do provide helpful information, many of them tend to promote sex as a purely technical and therefore less human activity. This technical approach to sex has the advantage of allowing private learning, but it permits men to remain in control by appearing to solve difficult human problems within a typical masculine framework which values logic and concrete results (Farrell, 1974).

Like some other aspects of the traditional male role, needs for power and control have important negative effects on heterosexual relationships. When men occupy the role of expert, teacher, initiator, leader, pleasure-giver, and so forth, women are deprived of experiencing the positive aspects of these roles; moreover, men deprive themselves of positively experiencing complementary roles which involve relaxing and receiving pleasure. Thus, the consequences of male sexual control limit female as well as male experience. For example, when men assume the knowledgeable teacher role, women frequently assume a complementary naive learner role. It is not difficult to extend the findings of Komarovsky's (1946) classic study (demonstrating that women sometimes feigned inferior performances with men in such activities as spelling and sailing) to sexual activities.

Ironically, Carlson's (1976) survey indicates that men are not altogether happy with their wives' sexually receptive follower role; these men desired "greater [sexual] participation on the part of their wives." Additional evidence of male dissatisfaction with the confines of the leader role is provided by Stein (1974) who systematically observed more than 1200 men in sexual interactions with call girls. Stein reports that the men frequently asked the call girl to direct the sexual activity. More than 10% of the middle-class clients in the Stein study evidenced a general sexual pattern which might be interpreted as a rebellion against the prescribed male role. These men, termed "slaves," asked the call girl to act out dominance/submission fantasies with them. Stein summarizes these data, "For many men, one of the attractions of the call girl seemed to be that with her they were not obligated to act out the traditionally 'masculine' role" (p. 45).

Because women have become increasingly aware of some of the limiting effects of male sexual control, men are more likely to encounter female partners who do take sexual initiative, assert sexual preferences, and complain when their needs are not considered or satisfied. A number of writers (Komarovsky, 1976; Safilios-Rothschild, 1977; Davies & Fisher, 1974) have commented on how the loss of sexual control has threatened men. One of the most highly touted effects of the recent shift away from male control is the so-called "new impotence," a term introduced by

Ginsberg, Frosch, and Shapiro (1972) and popularized by Nobile (1972). The Ginsberg et al. claim that there has been a notable increase in impotence especially among younger men is not supported by appropriate statistical comparisons—it may be that a large percentage of men have always suffered from impotence, or that men are simply more willing to report impotence today. Nonetheless it is plausible that men with a history of genital focus, sexual selfishness, sexual control and initiative now confronted with a new, more egalitarian set of rules may indeed be prone to impotence. Jayaratne (Note 5) reports that 54% of a youngish, highly educated sample of men (Tavris & Pope, 1976; Tavris, 1977) indicated they had experienced impotence, although three-fourths of this 54% said impotence occurred only "rarely." Very recent data (Pietropinto & Simenauer, 1977) from a reasonably representative sample of 4000 men indicate that 85% admitted a "potency problem at one time or another." Ginsberg and his psychiatric colleagues lay the blame for this state on the women's liberation movement and on the demands of individual women for increased sexual pleasure. In the context of this discussion, however, it seems more appropriate generally to attribute "new" male impotence to the restrictive socialization and sex typing which has made it difficult for men to relinquish control, to accept and enjoy less structured and more egalitarian sexual relationships.

AGGRESSION AND VIOLENCE

Although there has been some controversy about the extent of biological influence on aggression in the human male (Berkowitz, 1975), there is agreement that in Western culture at least, manliness is highly associated with forcefulness, aggression, and violence. It is no accident that there are few female football players, even fewer female boxers, and no female counterpart to John Wayne.

Many analyses linking male aggression and sexuality stem from Freudian energy concepts or from the configuration of the male and female genitalia themselves. An analysis which typifies both approaches is offered by Reik (1960):

> It should not be denied that the sexual urge of the male has an aggressive and even a sadistic character, and the wish to intrude the female body amounts to a kind of forceful incursion . . . the opening and invasion of another territory belongs to the realm of forepleasure comparable to that of forcing a door. The gradual extension and yielding of the female genitals enhances the enjoyment . . . Freud pointed out to us that one of the first manifestations of the sexual drive in adolescent boys is a wish to throw stones in windows and similar symptoms. Even the sexual curiosity of small boys has this aggressive, intrusive character [p. 118].

Probably the most extreme sexual manifestation of male aggression is rape. A number of writers (Brownmiller, 1975; Medea & Thompson, 1974; Russell, 1975) view rape as less an aberrant criminal act than a natural outgrowth of traditional male socialization. Russell, whose analysis is based on accounts of rape by rapists and their victims, suggests:

> [Rape] may be understood as an extreme acting out of the qualities that are regarded as supermasculine in this and many other societies: aggression, force, power, strength, toughness, dominance, competitiveness . . . sex may be the arena where those notions of masculinity are most intensely acted out, particularly by men who feel powerless in the rest of their lives [p. 260].

Russell succinctly summarizes her hypothesis in syllogistic form: "Being aggressive is masculine; being sexually aggressive is masculine; rape is sexually aggressive behavior; therefore rape is masculine behavior" (p. 261).

A similar oversocialization explanation is suggested by Weis and Borges (1973) who attribute sexual offenses to the link between traditional manliness and aggression: "The man by social convention is the initiator of sexual activity. Male zealots who oversubscribe to the masculine role image may combine hostile components of aggression with sexuality in an attempt to intimidate and dominate the female and thus validate their own identity" (p. 85). Griffin (1971) reasons that the norm for forceful sexual initiation, coupled with traditional social and legal views of woman as an extension or possession of man, provides a setting in which some men can justify "taking what is theirs" by force.

Because only a small percentage of men actually commit rape, and even fewer are brought to trial and convicted, there has been a tendency to view sexual aggression as a relatively limited phenonemon applying only to rapists and their victims. A series of interview studies by Eugene Kanin provides a sobering counterpoint to the comforting belief that heterosexual sex offenses are perpetrated only by a small population of deviant criminals. Offenses committed even by males of above average education are so pervasive that in one study (Kanin, 1965) more than 25% of the male undergraduate respondents admitted at least one incident of "sex aggression" since entering college. Sex aggression in this study was defined as a self-reported forceful attempt at coitus that resulted in the victim reacting by "crying, fighting, screaming, pleading, and so forth" (p. 221). In another study (Kirkpatrick & Kanin) more than half of 291 college women interviewed reported themselves "offended at least once during the academic year at some level of erotic intimacy" and 6% had experienced menacing threats or physical pain during the course of these offenses.

Not only is sexual aggression extremely common, but contrary to the popular notion that it occurs almost exclusively among strangers, Kanin (1957) reports that the most violent acts were even more likely to occur in the context of long-term relationships; and of course violence is not unknown in marriage, as attested to by the growing number of crisis centers to serve battered wives (Gingold, 1976).

As noted earlier, Kanin (1967) has stressed the role of male peer support for seduction and conquest, but in some instances "physical aggression and the resulting fear aroused in the female victim would (also) be applauded by college males" (1970, p. 35). Such aggression is usually justified by characterizing female victims as "golddiggers" and "cockteasers" who may be justly punished for their norm-violative behavior, or as promiscuous individuals who can be compelled to provide sexual services (Kanin, 1969). Both Kanin (1957) and Russell (1975) point out that heterosexual aggression may be encouraged by male fantasies that are commonly portrayed in the media. A dangerous prototype of this sort occurs in Peckinpaugh's violent film, *Straw Dogs,* in which a female rape victim valiantly resists for a few moments before acquiescing and ultimately responding ardently to her attacker. Selkin (1975) provides some evidence that these fantasies are sometimes translated into violent action. He reports that some convicted rapists insist that their victims enjoy sexual assault. Along these lines, Russell (1975), related this account of a rape: "Her date finally succeeded in raping her after a two-hour struggle, but he could not understand why she was so upset. . . . He considered himself a lover in the tradition of forceful males and expected to have a continuing relationship with her" (p. 258). In milder form, many women can attest to the sometimes unconscious confusion of sex and aggression that emerges in the many forms of "normal" male heterosexual activity.

Although peers probably reward men more for charming and manipulating women into bed than for coercing sex from female victims, it is likely that the overwhelming pressure on men to prove their masculinity via sexual performance indirectly leads to aggression and rape. Kanin (1970) reports that college peer groups, especially fraternities, "stress the erotic goal to such a degree that, in the face of sexual failure, there is a resorting to physical aggression" (p. 35).

The destructive consequences of male aggression for heterosexual relationships are a great deal less subtle than effects of some other facets of the male role. Most couples would agree, in theory at least, that mutual consent is a minimal prerequisite for good sexual relations; an intimidated or fearful woman can hardly be expected to engage in open communication, sexual or otherwise, with a physically stronger and potentially violent mate.

Other Influences

The aspects of the male sex role discussed above do not represent an exhaustive set of influences on sexual attitudes and behavior. There are undoubtedly many other consequences of the male socialization process which affect heterosexual relations, in fact most sex differences which have implications for social interaction also have implications for sexual interaction. One example of such a sex difference is that males typically report less general emotional expression (Allen & Haccoun, 1976), and they specifically report fewer expressions of love and happiness than females (Balswick & Avertt, 1977). Balswick and Peek (1971) have termed this male inexpressiveness "a tragedy of American society," and although "tragedy" may seem hyperbolic, it can be reasonably assumed that male failure to express positive emotion seriously impedes successful and rewarding communication with female sex partners for whom emotion and sex are inseparable concomitants.

TRADITIONAL AND MODERN MALE SEX ROLES

At the outset, I noted that although attempts to identify a definitive male sex role have proven frustrating, it is possible to isolate a number of typical male attitudes and behavior patterns and apply them to male sexuality. The approach of isolating these patterns may have implied that these typically masculine elements cannot be organized and labelled into more general syndromes or roles. This is clearly not the case; in the popular literature there presently exist at least two popularly held but contradictory characterizations of heterosexual man:

1. Man as exploitative sexual animal, an insensitive user of women, constantly on the prowl, grasping at any sexual opportunity, and gratifying himself quickly with little if any real caring or feeling for his partner.
2. Man as technically competent lover who strives to create multiple orgasmic pleasure for his partner; he asks, or better even senses, what she wants and then endeavors to provide it in his undaunting efforts to satisfy her.

The second, apparently more sensitive characterization has gained prominence in the past few years. Although the evolution from animal to technician (reflected and influenced by the proliferation of modern sex manuals, and perhaps best chronicled in the *Playboy* Advisor column) may at first appear egalitarian and progressive, it can be argued that this shift is basically a superficial one, and in any event largely restricted to the middle class (Rainwater, 1965; Rubin, 1976; Pleck, 1976). It should be obvious from the foregoing discussion that mechanical, unidimensional sex and success-oriented love-making both have their roots in the same sex-typed learning process, with similar pernicious effects.

In making a general distinction between modern and traditional sex roles, Pleck (1976) argues that the modern role has not served as a panacea for heterosexual ills; in fact it has brought with it a host of new problems.

Using a sexual example, Pleck (Note 6) discusses the shift from the traditional male goal of numerous sexual acts with many women to the more modern goal of sexually satisfying at least one woman. Both goals are quantitative: number of conquests in the former case, number of orgasms in the latter. Pleck points out that, like most general changes in the male role, this shift in sexual emphasis is a mixed blessing. On the one hand there may be a beneficial reduction in male predatory behavior, but on the other hand the creation of high sexual-performance standards for men has led to the use of concepts such as frigidity to blame women when men fail to satisfy them. Rubin (1976) captures the essence of a related modern problem in an interview with one of several wives in her sample who were preoccupied with their own orgasms "primarily because their husbands' sense of manhood rested on it":

> It's really important for him that I reach a climax and I try to every time. He says it just doesn't make him feel good if I don't. But it's hard enough to do it once! What'll happen if he finds out about those women who have lots of climaxes [p. 92]?

While few contemporary couples retain nostalgia for the days when men could efficiently "exercise marital rights" rather than "make love," it is apparent that the modern male role with its focus on sexual competence has created a whole set of new problems for heterosexual relationships.

Biology, Socialization, Sex Roles, and Sex

A number of recent contributions to the sexual literature (Gagnon & Simon, 1973; Gagnon, 1977; Byrne, 1977; Rook & Hammen, 1977) have widened the attack on the once inviolate ties between biology and human sexual behavior. And, as the influence of biological forces and Freudian psychological determinism wanes in the bedroom, possibilities that men and women can constructively choose to change their sexual behavior increase. Although reviewers of general sex differences (Maccoby & Jacklin, 1974; Deaux, 1976) have apparently concluded that biology can be modified or even overwhelmed by socialization, we have also learned in recent years that sex-typed learning experiences can build barriers as strong as those created by biology. But unlike the definitive pronouncements of the biologists, sex-role writings often contain a distinctly hopeful note that awareness of restrictions can lead to conscious and progressive change (for example, Deaux, 1976, p. 144). In this context, it is hoped that this discussion of the male sex role and its often destructive relationship to male sexual patterns will contribute to the understanding and eventually to the amelioration of negative heterosexual patterns for men and for the women with whom they relate.

68   *Theoretical Articles*

1. Crain, S., & Roth, S. *Interactional and interpretive processes in sexual initiation in married couples*. Paper presented at the meeting of the American Psychological Association, San Francisco, August 1977.
2. Rytting, M. B. *Sex or intimacy: Male and female versions of heterosexual relationships*. Paper presented at the meeting of the Midwestern Psychological Association, Chicago, May 1976.
3. Sanders, J. S. *Female and male language in communication with sexual partners*. Paper presented at the meeting of the Association for Women in Psychology, St. Louis, February 1977.
4. Skovholt, T. M., Nagy, F., & Epting, F. *Teaching sexuality to college males*. Paper presented at the meeting of the American Psychological Association, Washington, D.C., August 1976.
5. Jayaratne, T. Personal communication, November 1976.
6. Pleck, J. H. Personal communication, August 1976.

Allen, B. Liberating the manchild. *Transactional Analysis Journal*, 1972, *2*, 68–71.
Allen, J. G., & Haccoun, D. M. Sex differences in emotionality: A multidimensional approach. *Human Relations*, 1976, *29*, 711–722.
Balswick, J., & Avertt, C. P. Differences in expressiveness: Gender, interpersonal orientation, and perceived parental expressiveness as contributing factors. *Journal of Marriage and the Family*, 1977, *39*(1), 121–127.
Balswick, J., & Peek, C. The inexpressive male: A tragedy of American society. *The Family Coordinator*, 1971, *20*, 363–368.
Bardwick, J. M. Psychological conflict and the reproductive system. In J. M. Bardwick, E. Douvan, M. S. Horner, & D. Gutmann (Eds.), *Feminine personality and conflict*. Monterey, Calif,: Brooks/Cole, 1970.
Bardwick, J. M. *Psychology of women*. New York: Harper & Row, 1971.
Bem, S. L. The measurement of psychological androgyny. *Journal of Consulting and Clinical Psychology*, 1974, *72*, 155–162.
Bengis, I. *Combat in the erogenous zone*. New York: A. A. Knopf, 1972.
Berkowitz, L. *A survey of social psychology*. Hinsdale, Ill.: Dryden Press, 1975.
Brannon, R. The male sex role: Our culture's blueprint of manhood, and what it's done for us lately. In D. S. David & R. Brannon (Eds.), *The forty-nine percent majority: The male sex role*. Reading, Mass.: Addison-Wesley, 1976.
Broverman, I. K., Broverman, D. M., Clarkson, F. E., Rosenkrantz, P. S., & Vogel, S. R. Sex-role stereotypes and clinical judgments of mental health. *Journal of Consulting Psychology*, 1972, *34*, 1–7.
Brownmiller, S. *Against our will*. New York: Simon & Schuster, 1975.
Byrne, D. Social psychology and the study of sexual behavior. *Personality and Social Psychology Bulletin*, 1977, *3*, 3–30.
Carlson, J. E. The sexual role. In F. I. Nye (Ed.), *Role structure and analysis of the family*. Beverly Hills, Calif.: Sage Publications, 1976.
Davies, N. H., & Fisher, A. Liberated sex: The rise and fall of male potency. *Marriage and Divorce*, 1974, *1*(1), 66–69.

Deaux, K. *The behavior of women and men.* Monterey, Calif.: Brooks/Cole, 1976.

Farrell, W. *The liberated man: Beyond masculinity.* New York: Random House, 1974.

Fasteau, M. F. *The male machine.* New York: McGraw-Hill, 1974.

Freud, S. *Sexuality and the psychology of love.* New York: Macmillan (Collier Books), 1963. (Originally published, 1905.)

Gagnon, J. *Human sexualities.* Glenview, Ill.: Scott, Foresman, 1977.

Gagnon, J., & Henderson, B. *Human sexuality: An age of ambiguity.* Boston: Educational Associates, 1975.

Gagnon, J., & Simon, W. *Sexual conduct: The social sources of sexuality.* Chicago: Aldine, 1973.

Gingold, J. One of these days—Pow! Right in the kisser: The truth about battered wives. *Ms.*, 1976, *5*(2) 51–54; 94.

Ginsberg, G. L., Frosch, W. A., & Shapiro, T. The new impotence. *Archives of General Psychiatry,* 1972, *26*, 218–220.

Griffin, S. Rape: The all-American crime. *Ramparts,* 1971, *10*(3), 26–35.

Guinsburg, P. F. *An investigation of the components of platonic and romantic heterosexual relationships.* (Doctoral dissertation, University of North Dakota, 1973). (University Microfilms No. 73–39, 623.)

Hunt, M. Today's man. *Redbook,* October 1976, 112–113; 163–170.

Julty, S. A case of "sexual dysfunction." *Ms.*, 1972, *1*(4), 18–21.

Kaats, G. R., & Davis, K. E. The social psychology of sexual behavior. In L. S. Wrightsman (Ed.), *Social psychology in the seventies.* Monterey, Calif.: Brooks/Cole, 1972.

Kanin, E. J. Male aggression in dating-courtship relations. *American Journal of Sociology,* 1957, *63*, 197–204.

Kanin, E. J. Male sex aggression and three psychiatric hypotheses. *Journal of Sex Research,* 1965, *1*, 221–231.

Kanin, E. J. Reference groups and sex conduct norm violations. *The Sociological Quarterly,* 1967, *8*, 495–504.

Kanin, E. J. Selected dyadic aspects of male sex aggression. *Journal of Sex Research,* 1969, *5*.

Kanin, E. J. Sex aggression by college men. *Medical Aspects of Human Sexuality,* September 1970, 28–40.

Kinsey, A., Pomeroy, W. B., & Martin, C. E. *Sexual behavior in the human male.* Philadelphia: W. B. Saunders, 1948.

Kirkpatrick, C., & Kanin, E. Male sex aggression on a university campus. *American Sociological Review,* 1957, *22*, 52–58.

Koedt, A. *The myth of the vaginal orgasm.* Somerville, Mass.: New England Free Press, 1970.

Komarovsky, M. Cultural contradictions and sex roles. *American Journal of Sociology,* 1946, *52*, 182–89.

Komarovsky, M. *Dilemmas of masculinity: A study of college youth.* New York: Norton, 1976.

Korda, M. *Male chauvinism: How it works.* New York: Random House, 1973.

Landers, A. One boy's view of sex. *St. Louis Post-Dispatch,* May 29, 1976.

Maccoby, E. E., & Jacklin, C. N. *The psychology of sex differences.* Stanford, Calif.: Standford University Press, 1974.

Masters, W. H., & Johnson, V. E. *Human sexual response.* Boston: Little, Brown, 1966.

Masters, W. H., & Johnson, V. E. *Human sexual inadequacy*. Boston: Little, Brown, 1970.

McKee, J. P., & Sherriffs, A. C. The differential evaluation of males and females. *Journal of Personality*, 1957, *25*, 356–371.

Medea, A., & Thompson, K. *Against rape*. New York: Farrar, Straus, & Giroux, 1974.

Nichols, J. *Men's liberation: A new definition of masculinity*. New York: Penguin Books, 1975.

Nobile, P. What is the new impotence, and who's got it? *Esquire*, 1972, *78*(4), 95–98.

Peplau, L. A., Rubin, Z., & Hill, C. T. Sexual intimacy in dating relationships. *Journal of Social Issues*, 1977, *33* (2), 86–109.

Pietropinto, A., & Simenauer, J. *Beyond the male myth: What women want to know about men's sexuality*. New York: Times Books, 1977.

Pleck, J. H. The male sex role: Definitions, problems, and sources of change. *Journal of Social Issues*, 1976, *32* (3), 155–164.

Rainwater, L. Sexual and marital relations. In *Family Design*. Chicago: Aldine, 1965.

Reik, T. *Sex in men and women: Its emotional variations*. New York: Noonday Press, 1960.

Rook, K. S., & Hammen, C. L. A cognitive perspective on the experience of sexual arousal. *Journal of Social Issues*, 1977, *33*(2).

Rubin, L. *Worlds of pain: Life in the working class family*. New York: Basic Books, 1976.

Russell, D. E. H. *The politics of rape: The victim's perspective*. New York: Stein & Day, 1975.

Rytting, M. B. *Self-disclosure in the development of a heterosexual relationship*. Unpublished doctoral dissertation, Purdue University, 1975.

Safilios-Rothschild, C. *Love, sex and sex roles*. Englewood Cliffs, N.J.: Prentice-Hall, 1977.

Sawyer, J. On male liberation. *Liberation*, 1970, *15*, 32–33.

Selkin, J. Rape. *Psychology Today*, 1975, *8*(8), 70–72; 74–76.

Sheehy, G. *Passages: Predictable crises of adult life*. New York: Dutton, 1976.

Singer, M. Sexism and male sexuality. *Issues in Radical Therapy*, 1976, *3*, 11–13.

Stein, M. L. *Lovers, friends, slaves*. New York: Berkeley Publishing Co., 1974.

Tavris, C. Woman and man. In C. Tavris (Ed.), *The female experience*. Del Mar, Calif.: CRM Publishing Company, 1973.

Tavris, C. Men and women report their views on masculinity. *Psychology Today*, 1977, *10*(8), 34–42; 82.

Tavris, C., & Pope, D. Masculinity: What does it mean to be a man? *Psychology Today*, October 1976, 59–63.

Tharp, R. G. Dimensions of marriage roles. *Marriage and Family Living*, 1963, *25*, 389–404.

Weis, K., & Borges, S. S. Victimology and rape: The case of the legitimate victim. *Issues in Criminology*, 1973, *8*, 71–115.

Male
Homosexuality

JOSEPH L. NORTON
State University of New York at Albany

Being homosexual requires a good deal of adjustment, even in current times. Some homosexuals do quite well (Freedman, 1975), some do not (Bieber, Dain, Dince, Drellich, Grand, Gundlach, Kremer, Rifkin, Wilbur, & Bieber, 1962). Thus, any publication dealing with counseling men should explore the issues of being homosexual, as counselors and social scientists have been trained in the same myths and misinformation which have made life for the homosexual so difficult.

DEFINITIONS

In a recent chapter on counseling homosexuals, Kennedy (1977) quotes varying definitions of homosexuality. The simplest definition is "one who has an affectional and sexual preference for a person of the same sex." This, in a sense, leaves the matter one of self-definition, avoiding the outsider's varying labeling. For some, an individual with no same-sex experiences but regular fantasies would be homosexual; for others, two males with a mutual goal of getting each other to reach an erotic climax would be homosexual. Since so many males respond sexually to pressure on the genitals or other external stimulation, it almost seems as if intent should be part of the definition as Bieber et al. (1962) recommended. However, a single homosexual experience or so does not make one a homosexual.

One can question if a noun or adjective should be used at all, as one's sexuality is not the only aspect of life. Perhaps it is best only to talk of homosexual behavior (including imagery as behavior). Perhaps some day society can acknowledge simply that humans are sexual beings who can develop a wide repertoire of related behaviors, depending on a myriad of complex factors (Greene & Greene, 1973; Smith & Smith, 1974). But whatever the terminology, the homosexual person generally does develop a homosexual identity. Many who have identified themselves as homosexuals use the term "gay" as a self-chosen, nonclinical term. Gays use this term in preference to the outsiders' terms: homo, faggot, queer, or pansy.

CAUSES

Many authors have seen homosexuality as a disease. Thompson (1964) wrote that it "may express fear of the opposite sex, fear of adult responsibility, the need to defy authority, or an attempt to cope with hatreds of or competitive attitudes towards members of one's own sex; it may represent a flight from reality . . . or it may be a symptom of destructiveness of oneself or others." She does not see it representing love, affection, or a reaching out to an attractive love object, as many gays see it.

Homosexuality has been "blamed" on defective genes, defective hormone balances, defective parents (dominant mothers, absent or ineffectual fathers, dominant fathers), and inadequate training. The fact is that no one can say what causes it. Money and Ehrhardt (1972) and Shively and DeCecco (1977) discuss the development of sexual orientation and gender identity. (Sexual orientation means the type of person for whom an individual has an affectional and/or sexual preference; gender identity means the feeling a person has about what sex s/he is: male or female.) Both are complex; both seem to develop early in life, but there is no definitive cause of sexual orientation. The data are contradictory and most gays feel comfortable saying "You didn't do anything wrong" to their parents, whose first reaction to their son's declaration is negative.

When one considers the vast variety of people having same-sex orientation, the finding of a single cause seems improbable: the loving, monogamous young couple who met at a gay march, the old monogamous couple who met 35 years ago at church, the married man of the tearoom trade (Humphries, 1975), the divorced man who never wants to be tied down again, the newcomer to the bar scene who wants a new partner every night, the celibate priest, the closeted lawyer, the lawyer head of the Gay Community Center, the teacher, the drag queen, the hairdresser who flips his wrist, and the football player who doesn't. Actually, the list is endless. Gays are so varied it seems a waste to ask "why" and most gays don't care why, especially if the question is asked in the hopes of finding a "cure" or preventive. But, the "why" search will continue as long as there exists those who consider homosexuality an undesirable state.

Whatever the cause, same-sex orientation within the male is a very strong feeling that makes him overcome years and years of heterosexual upbringing and training so as to express who he believes he really is.

COMING OUT

The term "coming out" has different meanings. Fisher (1972) uses the term progressively to mean first, self-acceptance as a gay, then revelation to sexual partners, others in a gay rap group or gay bar, a trusted friend, selected family members, all family, then at school and/or church, work and perhaps finally to the general public. Lee (1977) on the other hand, discusses "going public" in three states: (1) self-identification and acceptance (signification), (2) coming out, or the "debut", and (3) going public. He feels that the "going public" stage is usually preceded by some involvement with a gay liberation group. Of course the examples given by some authors disagree with Lee (Miller, 1971). But whether or not one uses the term to cover all three of Lee's stages, some aspect of the process occurs in all males who eventually take on a homosexual lifestyle.[1]

As Lee points out, the first problem the gay male faces is acceptance of self. Many gay males report knowing they were different from age six on. Those who had early sexual experiences with peers felt they responded to this activity differently from their friends (who grew up to be nongay). Obviously, not all boys who feel "different" grow up to be homosexual, but many homosexuals knew early (unless one discounts these reports as selective remembering). Others do not discover themselves until their late teens, twenties, even fifties and sixties.

Without a positive role model, and with only the stereotype of the "visible" gay (the effeminate or drag-queen type), many homosexuals say "I'm not one of those," and spend years before they discover that there are others like themselves. Many others undergo extensive psychotherapy attempting to change that which they later come to enjoy (Brown, 1976; Reid, 1977; Smith, 1973). For the teenager, it is difficult. "Faggot" is the most degrading word in the typical American high school, and when you are one, you must work even harder to hide it (Brown, 1976; Kopay & Young, 1977; Reich, 1976; Reid, 1977).

How do gays know they are gay? They are attracted to other men; they fall in love with their "straight" roommates; they exhibit a greater sexual response to pictures of nude men than to those of nude women. They fantasize same-sex activity when masturbating and even when involved in heterosexual intercourse. However, anxiety about relationships with, or hatred for women does not seem to be characteristic of very many gays. According to one observer on the scene (Blair,1974), over 50% of

---

[1]The "straight" hustler who gets paid to be done by his trick is an example of how hard it is to come out; perhaps some of these men never acknowledge their homosexuality. But, one may ask, if they are not homosexual, why do they respond physically so readily? The classic heterosexual male would be so horrified as to be incapable of response.

male gays are heterosexually married; others report about 50% have had satisfactory heterosexual intercourse (Saghir & Robins, 1973; Weinberg & Williams, 1974).

Once the self-awareness stage has been accomplished, further steps in coming out are optional. Some remain inactive; others find a single partner to share both the secret and sex; others discover a gay subculture of bars and other meeting places; some find friends and through them, other friends, building a separate world; and, as indicated above, some become more and more open to others. Some find happiness, some do not—as is true of the heterosexual world.

OTHER STEREOTYPES AND MYTHS TO BE OVERCOME

It's Sick

"With the vote of the American Psychiatric Association, 20,000,000 Americans were cured" read one headline. Thus, "therapy by referendum" has helped somewhat to change attitudes, but the educational campaign that led to that two-to-one vote did not convince many, who base their views on the unhappy, visible homosexuals they have known in treatment. Would we take 106 couples from Masters and Johnson's clinic and write the definitive book on heterosexuality? The classic work by Bieber et al. (1962) was based only on homosexuals in treatment, yet ironically, the *Journal of Abnormal Psychology* was the source of an early article reporting that gays are as well adjusted (didn't use the work "normal") as heterosexuals (Thompson, McCandless, & Strickland, 1971). Freedman (1975) summarized many of these under the title "Gays May Be Healthier Than Straights." Horstman (1975) found that MMPI scores did not differentiate diagnostically between gays and straights.

Child Molestation

Statistics on crime clearly show that child molestation (besides being primarily a family matter) is 95% heterosexual, so the 10% of the population who are gay do not produce their proportional share. The idea that youngsters are seduced into homosexuality by their elders, although confirmed by individual cases, is contradicted by the data that most gay males have their first sex with someone within 3 years of their own age, and by Rossman's (1976) report that it is usually the youth who initiates adult-youth sexual activities once a friendly relationship is established.

Influence on Children by Positive Role Models

Anita Bryant's scare tactic "Would you want your child to be taught by one?" is based on no data at all. It is safe to say that almost all youth have been taught by homosexuals without turning gay; the *New York*

Times estimates 120,000 to 240,000 gay teachers; if they had all been recruiting, certainly the heterosexual world would have heard of it (Macroff, 1977). If people could be influenced by the sexual proclivities of their teachers, most of the older generation would, as it has been so tartly put, be spinsters; and most Catholic women, nuns. Certainly, if most extensive therapeutic (and punitive) efforts at changing homosexuals to heterosexuals fail, why is it logical to expect that the "pressure" of an openly gay teacher would turn youth into homosexuals!

Role Playing the Opposite Sex

This stereotype, again, seems to be based on the visible, effeminate homosexual, estimated to be 10 to 20% of the gay population (Lee, 1977, p. 75). Homosexual male couples no longer usually take on the "husband" and "wife", "provider" and "housekeeper" roles. Mutuality is reported to be the rule (Mombello, 1977; Gay Couple Counseling, 1974).

The Lonesome Aging Gay

Karlen (1971, p. 531) passes on this stereotype, of the lonesome sexless "auntie" as "a specter before the eyes of young homosexuals." The facts (Francher & Hankin, 1973; Kelly, 1977) belie the myth. Many older gays have lovers, or a circle of friends (for companionship or sex) to accompany their other interactions with the heterosexual world of work, church or other. While some older homosexuals have accepted this much-reported stereotype, their more active colleagues find such pessimism unnecessary (Kleinberg, 1977).

Other Myths

Most of the other myths, like gays wanting to be women and being very feminine, can be dispelled by any alert observer. David Kopay, the football player, is not a weak, introspective, physically inactive person. Gay baseball teams in San Francisco sometimes defeat the police teams. There are gay groups in almost all professions (law, medicine, anthropology, nursing, psychology, counseling, teaching—but not yet dentistry), so the fear that a gay has to be an artist, interior decorator, or hairdresser can be dispelled.

Since studies of transvestites and transsexuals (both pre-and post-operative) reveal that 80% of the former and virtually all of the latter see themselves as heterosexuals, the confusion of these people with the stereotypical gay male can be eliminated. So too can the fear that relaxing laws about same-sex sexual activity will cause an increase in homosexual activity. In the first seven of the 19 states that have removed their "sodomy statutes," there has been no increase in the involvement of homosexuals with minors, the use of force by homosexuals, or the amount of private homosexual behavior (Geis, Wright, Garrett, & Wilson, 1976).

THE COMPETENT HOMOSEXUAL

On a 1973 David Susskind show, six homosexuals appeared on a panel entitled "The Professional Gay Comes Out." Unlike the six who appeared a few years earlier with paper bags over their heads, these six gave names and positions. None lost his or her job or professional status, and in fact one was later elected to the Massachusetts State Legislature. The professional leaders of the various gay (and bi-) caucuses already mentioned, and the leaders of the gay caucuses in the major religious denominations of the country, as well as the gay activist leaders themselves attest to the fact that gays are to be found in every walk of life and can manage a homosexual life style in comfort. Since Hooker's (1967) initial study, other research has supported the notion that being homosexual is only part of life, and that gays have as many and varied competencies and capabilities (and faults) as heterosexuals (Freedman, 1975; Mombello, 1977).

HOMOPHOBIA

This term, a short form of homoerotophobia, is used by Weinberg (1972) to refer to an extreme fear of contact with homosexuals. That it exists can be attested to not only by the writer's house being set fire to, after a newspaper profile appeared, but also by studies (Karr, 1975; McConaghy, 1967; Morin, 1975; Smith, 1971). Its "causes" have been postulated as fear of the homosexual feelings inside one's self and a general rigidity and conservatism about life and sex (the authoritarian personality) (MacDonald & Games, 1974; Sherrill, 1974; Silverstein, 1973). One "straight" suggested a new one to the writer recently: jealousy—of the freedom, of the (stereotyped) promiscuity. Whatever its causes, it is a fairly rampant problem, and counselors and psychologists do not seem to be automatically immune. Yet it can be cured, and the best cure is extended exposure to some well-adjusted gays.

CONCLUSION

The material reviewed here does not seem to be saying there should be a "psychology of homosexuality." If psychologists viewed homosexuals as people just as they do heterosexuals, if society would take the pressures off the teenage gay, it would seem clear that homosexuals are (if a separate group at all), a group of people with an alternate life style, and an alternate love style. They have the same interpersonal problems the "straight" world has—communication problems, love, jealousy, fear of rejection, elation over successes. They have no better a future nor worse.

Until that "iffy" world comes to pass, there are some special problems facing the gay male in coming out. There are some special issues with which gays can be helped. how do I know if I'm gay; should I come out—how will my parents react; can I get a job; will I be able to leave my possessions to my lover; how much hassle will I get from a predominantly nongay world? Several articles address themselves more extensively to these questions than is possible here (Bernstein, 1977; Haynes, 1977; Jones, 1974; Norton, 1976, 1977).

REFERENCES

Bernstein, B. E. Legal and social interface in counseling homosexual clients. *Social Casework*, 1977, *58*, 36–40.
Bieber, I., Dain, H. J., Dince, P. R., Drellich, M. G., Grand, H. G., Gundlach, R. H., Kremer, M. W., Rifkin, A. H., Wilbur, C. B., & Bieber, T. B. *Homosexuality: A psychoanalytic study.* New York: Basic Books, 1962.
Blair, R. Personal communication, 1974.
Brown, H. *Familiar faces, hidden lives: The story of homosexual men in America today.* New York: Harcourt Brace Jovanovich, 1976.
Fisher, P. *The gay mystique: The myth and reality of male homosexuality.* New York: Stein & Day, 1972.
Francher, S., & Hankin, J. The menopausal queen: Adjustment to aging and the male homosexual. *American Journal of Orthopsychiatry,* 1973, *43*(4), 670–674.
Freedman, M. Homosexuals may be healthier than straights. *Psychology Today,* 1975, *8*(10), 28–32.
Gay couple counseling: Proceedings of a conference. *Homosexual Counseling Journal,* 1974, *1*, 88–139.
Geis, G., Wright, R., Garrett, T., & Wilson, P. R. Reported consequences of decriminalization of consensual adult homosexuality in seven American states. *Journal of Homosexuality,* 1976, *1*, 419–426.
Greene, G., & Greene, C. *S-M, the last taboo.* New York: Grove Press, 1973.
Haynes, A. The challenge of counseling the homosexual client, *Personnel and Guidance Journal,* 1977, *56*(4), 243–246.
Hooker, E. The adjustment of the male overt homosexual. *Journal of Projective Techniques,* 1957, *21*, 18–31.
Horstman, W. R. MMPI responses of homosexual and heterosexual male college students. *Homosexual Counseling Journal,* 1975, *2*(2), 68–76.
Humphries, L. *The tearoom trade: Impersonal sex in public places* (Rev.ed.). Chicago: Aldine Press, 1975.
Jones, C. R. *Homosexuality and counseling.* Philadelphia: Fortress Press, 1974.
Karlen, A. *Sexuality and homosexuality, a new view.* New York: Norton, 1971.
Karr, R. *Homosexual labeling: An experimental study.* Paper presented at Western Psychological Association convention, Sacramento, April 1975.
Kelly, J. The aging male homosexual: Myth and reality. *The Gerontologist,* 1977, *17*, 328–332.
Kennedy, E. *Sexual counseling.* New York: Seabury Press, 1977.
Kleinberg, S. Those dying generations: Harry and his friends. *Christopher Street,* 1977, *2*(5), 6–26.
Kopay, D., & Young, P. D. *The David Kopay story.* New York: Arbor House, 1977.

Lee, J. A. Going public: A study in the sociology of homosexual liberation. *Journal of Homosexuality*, 1977, *3*, 49–78.

MacDonald, A. P., Jr., & Games, R. G. Some characteristics of those who hold positive and negative attitudes toward homosexuals. *Journal of Homosexuality*, 1974, *1*, 9–27.

Macroff, G. I. Should professed homosexuals be permitted to teach school? *New York Times*, June 24, 1977.

McConaghy, N. Penile volume change to moving pictures of male and female nudes in heterosexual and homosexual males. *Behavior Therapy and Research*, 1967, *5*, 43–48.

Miller, M. *On being different: What it means to be a homosexual.* New York: Random House, 1971.

Mombello, R. *To come out, an alternative for the young male homosexual.* Laguna Beach, Calif.: Author, 1977.

Money, J., & Ehrhardt, A. *Man and woman, boy and girl.* Baltimore: Johns Hopkins Press, 1972.

Morin, S. *Attitudes toward homosexuality and social distance.* Paper presented at the American Psychological Association convention, Chicago, September 1975.

Norton, J. L. The homosexual and counseling. *Personnel and Guidance Journal*, 1976, *54*(7), 374–377.

Norton, J. L. Counseling on homosexuality. *Journal of Sex Education and Therapy*, 1977, *3*(2), 29–30.

Reich, C. *The sorcerer of Bolinas Reef.* New York: Random House, 1976.

Reid, J. *The best little boy in the world.* New York: Ballantine, 1977.

Rossman, P. *Sexual experience between men and boys.* New York: Association Press, 1976.

Saghir, M., & Robins, E. *Male and female homosexuality: A comprehensive investigation.* New York: Williams & Wilkins, 1973.

Sherrill, K. *Homophobia: Illness or disease?* Paper presented at American Political Science Association convention, New York City, August 1974.

Shively, G., & DeCecco, P. Components of sexual identity. *Journal of Homosexuality*, 1977, *3*, 41–48.

Silverstein, C. *Homophobia.* Paper presented at Gay Academic Union 1, New York, 1973.

Smith, A. Statement on the David Susskind show, 1973.

Smith, J. R., & Smith, L. G. *Beyond monogamy.* Baltimore: Johns Hopkins Press, 1974.

Smith, K. Homophobia: A tentative personality profile. *Psychological Reports*, 1971, *29*, 1091–1094.

Thompson, C. *Interpersonal psychoanalysis: The selected papers of Clara Thompson.* New York: Basic Books, 1964.

Thompson, N. L., McCandless, B. R., & Strickland, B. R. Personal adjustment of male and female homosexuals and heterosexuals. *Journal of Abnormal Psychology*, 1971, *78*, 237–240.

Weinberg, G. *Society and the healthy homosexual.* New York: St. Martins Press, 1972.

Weinberg, M. S., & Williams, C. J. *Male homosexuals: Their problems and adaptations.* New York: Oxford University Press, 1974.

Emotional Intimacy among Men

ROBERT A. LEWIS
Arizona State University

Although males report more same-sex friendships than women do, most of these are not close, intimate, or characterized by self-disclosure. Many barriers exist to emotional intimacy between men, some stemming from the demands of traditional male roles in our society, such as pressures to compete, homophobia, and aversion to vulnerability and openness, as well as from the lack of adequate role models. Exercises to increase self-disclosure, openness, and the potential for deeper affection between men are described as the goals of workshops developed to enable male participants to initiate and maintain meaningful relationships with other men.

This article is not about sexual behavior between men, nor about typical male friendships; it is concerned with something in between—that is, emotional intimacy. Emotional intimacy is defined in behavioral terms as mutual self-disclosure and other kinds of verbal sharing, as declarations of liking or loving the other, and as demonstrations of affection such as hugging and nongenital caressing.

Cultural prohibitions in America, as well as in many other Western nations, frown strongly upon the demonstration of intimacy between men, such as adult males openly sharing affection in public. As a consequence, many American males in adult life have never had a close male friend nor known what it means to love and care for a male friend without the shadow of some guilt and fear of peer ridicule (Komarovsky, 1974; Pleck, 1975a; Goldberg, 1976). Because of these restrictive norms, even those who have male friends usually have experienced little trust, little personal sharing, and low emotional investments in these friendships (Jourard, 1971; Fasteau, 1972, 1974; Steinmann & Fox, 1974; Pleck, 1974, 1975a; Goldberg, 1976). There is more than a little irony in the keen observation that many

"Emotional Intimacy Among Men," by R. A. Lewis, *Journal of Social Issues,* 1978 *34*(1), 108–121. Copyright 1978 by the Society for the Psychological Study of Social Issues. Reprinted by permission.

Correspondence regarding this article may be addressed to R. A. Lewis, Center for Family Studies, Arizona State University, Tempe, AR 85281.

American men report their closest male relationships as those discovered through war or sports—that is, when they are bonded together to kill others (Fasteau, 1974).

Don Clark, a psychologist who has worked frequently with all-male groups, has reflected that:

> Men need more from one another than they believe they are permitted to have. Expression of positive affect, or affection, between men is seriously inhibited in our culture. Negative affect is acceptable. Men can argue, fight, and injure one another in public view, but they cannot as easily hold hands, embrace, or kiss. When emotions in any area are blocked in expression, they seek other outlets, in distorted form if necessary [1972, p. 368].

DEFICITS IN EMOTIONAL INTIMACY

Research on male friendships suggests that most males are not very emotionally intimate with other males. Two studies (Olstad, 1975; Powers & Bultena, 1976) suggest that, although men may report more same-sex friendships than women do, these friendships are not close or intimate. For instance, Olstad's study of Oberlin college students reported that the majority of Oberlin males had more male best friends than female best friends. Yet these males tended to place greater confidence in, consulted more about important decisions, and spent more time together with their best female friends than with their best male friends. Powers and Bultena (1976) in a statewide study in Iowa interviewed 234 noninstitutionalized adults who were 70 years or older. Their findings suggested that the aged males had more frequent social contacts than did the aged females, but that the males basically limited their social interaction to their children and their children's families, and to spouses. The aged men also were less likely than the women to have intimate friends and were less likely to replace their lost friends.

Similar findings have been discussed by Knupfer, Clark, and Room (1966), who found unmarried males to have less close relationships with both sexes than females had. Finally, Nye (1976) reported that married men also went less to same-sex and other-sex friends for "therapeutic" purposes than their wives did.

Self-disclosure, a vital component of emotional intimacy, has been reported in many studies to be either very low or utterly lacking between males (Jourard, 1971). Similarly, in Komarovsky's survey of males at an Ivy League college (1974, 1976), college males disclosed themselves much more to their closest female friend than to their closest male friend. For most men, apparently, it is difficult and embarrassing to tell one's best male friend that he is liked. A recent nationwide survey (Pleck, Note 1) reported that a majority—58% of all males questioned—had not told their best male friend that they liked him. If the disclosure of liking one another is so difficult, it is little wonder that hugging, holding hands, caressing and kissing, which are allowed between close male friends in some cultures, are not often observed in our own culture.

The lack of emotional intimacy between men is currently being decried from a number of quarters. Some writers have even taken the position that the absence of intimate behavior among men is a microcosm spreading to many social problems. Goldberg (1976) argues that the absence of a loving, close male relationship is strongly related to the significantly higher suicide rates among males, especially among divorced males. The Berkeley Men's Center Manifesto (1973), perhaps the first declaration of men's liberation, contains these words:

> We, as men, want to take back our full humanity. . . . We want to relate to both women and men in more human ways—with warmth, sensitivity, emotion, and honesty. We want to share our feelings with one another to break down the walls and grow closer. We want to be equal with women and end destructive, competitive relationships between men. . . . We are oppressed by this dependence on women for support, nurturing, love, and warm feelings. We want to love, nurture, and support ourselves and other men, as well as women. . . . We want men to share their lives and experiences with each other in order to understand who we are, how we got this way, and what we must do to be free.

In a similar voice, Pleck and Sawyer have stated:

> Many of us are still working out in our own lives just what degree of emotional and sexual intimacy we want with others, both male and female. However each of us works this out, many of us already know that the traditional masculine role allows much less emotional expression with other males than we want, and that we must seek more [1974, p. 75].

BARRIERS TO INTIMACY BETWEEN MEN

Competition

A number of recent essays have traced some of the barriers to male intimacy to norms prescribed by American society (Fasteau, 1974; Pleck, 1974, 1975b; Brannon, 1976; Goldberg, 1976). Pleck (1975b), for instance, attributes much affectional inhibition among men to our society's stress upon competition—what Brannon (1976) has called the ''Big Wheel'' dimension of the traditional male sex role. Pleck traces a number of ancient, as well as contemporary, fables about male/male relationships that have prescribed a heavy component of competition even among friends. In fact, he suggests that, since many ''power trips'' are directed toward other men, in order to win more approval, wealth, and status, it is very difficult for male friends to mutually disclose themselves, since disclosure amounts to increased vulnerability in a competitive milieu.

There is some empirical evidence that male children realize at an early age that part of being a man is to compete and win. Hartley (1959), for instance, suggested that her sample of 41 boys between the ages of 8–11 understood clearly that a man "is supposed to be rugged, independent, able to take care of himself, and to disdain 'sissies' . . . [that] they have to be able to fight in case a bully comes along; they have to be athletic; they have to be able to run fast; they must be able to play rough games; they need to know how to play many games—curb-ball, baseball, basketball, football" (p. 460.)

Vinacke (1959), with the backing of evidence from several experimental studies, concludes that "males are primarily concerned with winning, whereas females are more oriented towards working out an equitable outcome, as satisfactory as possible to all participants" (p. 359). In another study, Vinacke and Gullickson (1964) asked triads of same-sex subjects from ages 7 to 8, 14 to 16, and college students to play a game similar to Parcheesi through which they could operationalize competition/exploitation as well as cooperative/accommodative behavior. They concluded:

> Girls at all three age levels display the characteristics of accommodative strategy. Boys, however, appear to change drastically from behavior quite similar to that of girls to the contrasting strategy which we have called "exploitative." Competitiveness . . . such behavior so typical of adult males, appears to exist only in rudimentary form in small boys [1229].

Finally, Szal (1972) reported that, while pairs of females took turns in playing games of marbles so that each won an equal number of times, pairs of males competed so strongly that neither could win many games.

Clearly, it is hard to reach out affectionately to other males beyond a superficial level if one views all males as competitors in life. Komarovsky (1974) frequently noted college males suggesting that learning to let down their guard and trust other men came with great difficulty, since they had been taught to be alert for aggressive attacks even from their friends:

> The main disadvantage of a male friend, as confidant, was his threat as a competitor. "A guy means competition." One senior explained: "I have competed with guys in sports and for girls. Once you let your guard down, the guy can hurt you and take advantage of you. Your girl has your interest at heart." "Even your best (male) friend," remarked one senior wryly, "gets a certain amount of comfort out of your difficulty. A girl friend is readier to identify with your interests and to build you up" [p. 680].

In sum, competition, which is prescribed by the traditional male role, is a barrier to intimacy between men. As DeGolia (1973) has written: "men are kept isolated from each other through competition and fear" (p. 16). And as Verser (Note 2) has commented: "since a main form of winning is exploiting the opponent's weaknesses, men close themselves off from each other, so that they do not expose any vulnerabilities."

Homophobia

Another barrier to intimacy between men is homophobia. Homophobia, the fear of homosexuals or the fear of one's being or appearing to be homosexual, is still very strong within our culture; this is especially the case for males. This barrier to intimacy stems from both conscious and unconscious fears that any intimacy between men may color one's sexual identity with gay colors.

It was homophobia that restricted the growth of affection between two friends in James Kirkwood's *P.S. Your Cat is Dead,* a play in which the hero relates:

> One evening about three months into our friendship, after we'd taken our dates home, we stopped by a bar for a nightcap. We ended up having three or four and when we left and were walking down the street, Pete suddenly slipped his arm around my shoulder. He surprised me; there was extreme warmth and intimacy about the gesture. When I looked over at him, he grinned as casual as possible. "Why?" He shrugged in return, then gave my shoulder a squeeze. "Ever since I've known you, you got me pretending I don't have arms" [1973, p. 23].

The fear of touching another male, unless it is roughly done as in a game of football or other contact sport, undoubtedly derives not only from strong cultural prohibitions against male homosexuality, but also from many Americans' difficulty or inability to distinguish between the sensual and the sexual.

Nearly all of the data on homophobia or negative attitudes toward homosexuality is correlational—that is, survey findings which relate personality, demographic, and other attitudes with homophobic attitudes. Morin and Garfinkle (1978), summarizing this research, report homophobia to be more characteristic of people who are likely also to be rural, White, male, first-born, reared in the Midwest and the South, more religious, and more conforming, with personality correlates that are more authoritarian, dogmatic, intolerant of ambiguity, status conscious, sexually rigid, guilty, and negative about their own sexual impulses, and less accepting of others in general. Nevertheless, Morin and Wallace (Note 3) found through a multiple regression analysis that the single best predictor of homophobia was a belief in the traditional family ideology where the father is dominant and the mother is subservient.

There is some evidence that homophobia operates to maintain social distance between gays and straights. For instance, Wolfgang and Wolfgang (1971) used the placement of stick figures to measure social distance and found subjects placing themselves significantly further from marijuana users, drug addicts, obese persons, and present and former homosexuals, than from "normal" peers. Similarly, Morin, Taylor, and Kielman (Note 4) found through the methodology of chair placement that males increased their social distance about three times more than did females where a male experimenter had been identified as a gay psychologist.

There is no experimental evidence to show that homophobia prevents emotional intimacy between heterosexual men, although such a connection has been long assumed (Pleck, 1975a). In fact, most writers on this subject seem to agree with Morin and Garfinkle (1978) that "the fear of being labeled homosexual . . . interferes with the development of intimacy between men."

Aversion to Vulnerability and Openness

Sexual stereotypes of males in the United States usually include some allusion to males being inexpressive or emotionally controlled. Bardwick and Douvan (1971) concluded that stereotypes of masculinity dictate that big boys are made of "aggression, competitiveness, task orientation, unsentimentality, and emotional control" (p. 225). Chafetz (1974) reports from group discussions of five to six undergraduate students that most Americans characterize males as "unemotional, stoic, and don't cry" (p. 35).

Brannon's (1976) characterization of American men as always having to be "the sturdy oak"—that is, having to maintain a "manly air of toughness, confidence, and self reliance"—indicates another barrier to male/male intimacy. If a man must never show any weaknesses even with his friends, he is under the additional burden of keeping secrets about his weaknesses, his errors, and his pains. The result of keeping these secrets is the "inexpressive male," as exemplified in the John Wayne "cowboy syndrome" and the James Bond "playboy syndrome," which have been well described by Balswick and Peek (1971). In fact, some men become so skilled in hiding their feelings and thoughts that even their wives and closest friends do not know when they are most depressed, anxious, or afraid.

Jourard's programmatic research on self-disclosure has documented the fact that males reveal much less personal information about themselves to others than do women (Jourard, 1971; Jourard & Lasakow, 1958; Jourard & Landsman, 1960; Jourard & Richman, 1963). Not only does the male aversion to vulnerability and openness handicap attempts to achieve emotional intimacy between men, but, as Jourard (1971) has suggested, always trying to be "manly" imposes a terrible burden upon many men, imposes extra stresses, consumes much personal energy, and consequently is a factor related to males' relatively shorter life span.

Lack of Role Models

A fourth barrier to the expression of emotional intimacy between men is the fact that many men have been presented few models or examples of affection-giving between males. In the course of a series of intimacy workshops that this author led between 1975 and 1977, more than half of the male participants have reported that they do not remember their fathers hugging them, especially after they were somewhat older children.

Although current films and books have probably portrayed friendships between males more often than between females, our popular culture is seemingly devoid of interest in male/male affection. Outside of homoerotic literature, there is little to guide men who are trying to share intimacy without sex. In a number of recent novels, men come close but do not find permission to give each other affection. For example, in *Deliverance* (Dickey, 1970) men in the wilderness are allowed to rape and murder each other but not share more than a canoe. In the novel *Radcliffe* (Storey, 1963), two boyhood friends eventually become involved in sexual intimacy, but apparently this must end "naturally" in the murder of one and the suicide of the other. A similar ending occurs for the young athlete in *The Front Runner* (Warren, 1974).

Although the barriers to male intimacy are undoubtedly more numerous than those described here, they illustrate well why most intimacy between males is confined in our culture to games that men can play together; for example, sports. As many current observers have noted, without a game to play, men usually do not relate well together.

THE TRADITIONAL MALE ROLE AND INTIMACY

Three of the four barriers to emotional intimacy between males stem directly from the traditional male role into which most men in our society have been socialized. That is to say, a male's acceptance of traditional male role expectations strongly reinforces his efforts to be competitive, to fear homosexuality, and to avoid personal vulnerability and openness, all of which make emotional intimacy between men more difficult to attain. The fourth barrier, the scarcity of role models, is more of a cyclical effect of male role performances from previous generations; these have been documented for middle-aged men by Steinmann and Fox (1974).

Several writers have related males' difficulties in establishing relationships to the pressures and demands of the male sex role (Fasteau, 1974; Pleck, 1974). Brannon (1976) examines four themes of traditional American masculitity ("no sissy stuff," "be a big wheel," "be the sturdy oak," and "give 'em hell'") and suggests similarly that they limit the development of meaningful relationships for men. Even earlier, Jourard (1971) had examined the "lethal aspects of the male role": the ways in which traditional expectations of manliness result for men in lower self-disclosure, a lack of self-insight and empathy, incompetence at loving others and self, and "dispiritation"—that is, the condition in which a man's morale and immunity to diseases decrease as a result of his not being able to live up to stringent masculine ideals.

A growing number of research findings appear to substantiate this linkage between the traditional male role and men's difficulties in relating to both women and other men. Mussen (1962) found that men who were more masculine in adolescence were rated twenty years later as less "sociable," less "self-assured," and less "self-accepting" than the men who had been less masculine in adolescence. Harford, Willis, and Deabler (1967) found a negative relationship also between traditional masculinity and "sensitivity" among men. The methodology of these earlier studies was limited to paper and pencil techniques. However, a recent experimental study by Bem, Martyna, and Watson (1976) has demonstrated that more masculine males have higher thresholds than either androgynous or more feminine males for displaying emotionality. Bem et al. found that the more masculine men were significantly less responsive to a male stranger who needed to talk about his loneliness and to be supported. An observational study of interaction patterns in same-sex groups (Aries, 1976) likewise suggested that men in all-male college groups were much less intimate and open than were women in all-female groups. In fact, the men talked very little of themselves, their feelings, or their relationships with significant others, whereas the women frequently did. It seems, therefore, that the sex-role demands of conventional American society powerfully limit the degree of intimacy that males may attain, especially in their relationships with other men.

INTIMACY WORKSHOP EXPERIENCES

Since 1975 I have conducted a number of workshops at men's conferences around the United States and Canada. The focus of these workshops has been the development of openness and intimacy between males. The increasing number of men who have been attracted to these workshops is some evidence that many men are desirous of closer relationships with other men.

Self-Disclosure

The first major objective in these workshops has been the opening of communication between men, most of whom are strangers. Working within small groups of two or three, the participants have been asked first to introduce themselves to one other person in the room and to tell as much about themselves as is possible within a ten-minute period. At the end of this time, each participant is then asked to introduce the other person to the larger group. The typical introduction involves a man's name, his occupation, his marital status, his residence, the number of his children if any, and sometimes even a list of his hobbies or leisure-time pursuits. All of these are predictable masculine disclosures, predictable because they involve the roles a man plays in society. In addition, the first disclosures are usually relatively "safe"—a fact that is quickly brought to the group's awareness, along with an appeal to risk more during the next group experience, such as telling things about themselves that they usually would tell only a very close friend.

Some risk taking usually proceeds with haste and is evident in the number of self-disclosures which are indicated, although not always shared with the entire group, during the second reporting period. About this time the intensity of the small group interaction usually breaks forth in very spontaneous and unpredictable fashion. In spite of the fact that the workshop is a relatively artificial social group of strangers, the breakthroughs in terms of self-disclosure are amazing. Participants have described later to us how for the first time in their life they were able to share thoughts and feelings about which they had never before spoken. One man described it this way:

> I have never even told my wife about that feeling I have often had. Now
> I cannot wait to get home and tell her. What a relief this is for me.

Self-disclosure is probably one of the most difficult forms of intimacy to initiate and facilitate between men. This is probably due to the fact that even as young boys, men have been taught to play it "cool and tough" (Hartley, 1959). No wonder that by the time most men are adults, they disclose much less about themselves than women do, especially to other males. And yet, we have found that many of the barriers to self-disclosure melt away in these workshops where permission is given to disclose oneself and one is surrounded by the acceptance and warm support of other men.

Extending Affection

A second series of exercises usually focuses upon the achievement of some physical intimacy, such as touching hands. In spite of many initial inhibitions, we have found most groups eager to be involved in a physical way. Although there are still signs of embarrassment and timidity for some men, most are able to complete the remaining intimacy exercises which involved further self-disclosure while touching or holding hands and looking directly into another man's eyes. The averting of eyes is another barrier to male intimacy (Argyle, 1967) which takes concerted efforts to break.

The greatest breakthroughs to demonstrating affection, however, usually are achieved through a larger group experience of affection. One of the most popular is the group hug, a configuration formed by men holding hands and winding themselves into a tight human coil. As some participants have related: "You lose contact of where you begin and end in the group hug," and "If this is what a football huddle feels like, I wish I had gone out for the varsity." An activity such as the group hug or any of the many trust exercises used in growth groups usually gives visual evidence of a sudden release from inhibitions which were still evident in the smaller dyadic and triadic groups. Whether this dynamic release from earlier inhibitions is due to the greater anonymity within the larger group or due to the total accumulation of experiences is not known. The final products, however, have been a proliferation of many spontaneous acts of intimacy witnessed throughout the room, amid laughing and hugging. Fairly common have been open-ended invitations by one or more of the participants, such as overt requests for the demonstration of affection. One typical comment has been: "I never get enough hugs, so, anyone who wants to hug me can." And, interestingly, not one of these invitations has ever been ignored.

COPING WITH INVITATIONS TO INTIMACY

One concern which has not yet risen in these workshops but which seems to be a problematic area voiced by individuals who are learning to be emotionally intimate is the question: how do males cope with unwanted invitations to intimacy? Also, how do I know the amount and type of intimacy that I wish from a male friend? Finally, how can I keep the intimacy to a level and kind that I also desire, that will not threaten other intimate relationships such as a marriage or other meaningful relationships with women? In particular, the opening of emotionally warm relationships between males may also involve the exposing of one's life to many new relationship problems, such as jealousy, rejection, and the fear of rejection.

Some men have experienced one or more of these problems firsthand in their early attempts at learning to relate to another male at a more intimate level. For instance, some have taken risks later in their ongoing friendships by honestly sharing their feelings of liking or loving. Fortunately, none of these revelations have been met with physical violence or reactions that have threatened these ongoing friendships.

Out of all possible reactions to overt male protestations of liking or loving one could envision the following points along an entire continuum of reactions: (a) physical violence or other hostile rejection—for example, the revealee beating up the revealor; (b) obvious repulsion experienced by the revealee toward revealor with subsequent attempts to avoid revealor; (c) no reaction, such as attempts to ignore the message and the sender or creating a momentary diversion so that revealee does not have to deal with an uncomfortable situation, (d) acceptance of the message with no reciprocity of similar feelings of love or liking; and (e) acceptance with reciprocity of similar prostestations.

The finding of most responses from my friends falling into category (d) perhaps tells more about my friends than about the process of coping with typical invitations to intimacy, since many are counselors and therapists who have learned to handle feelings of transference and counter-transference. However, that which my ethnomethodological experiments have thus far not taught is how to handle rejection from males. Upon entering the dating game in adolescence, men learn to cope with rejections by females. But how do men learn to cope with personal rejections by males? It may be that the male ego may prove too fragile or friendships too few to allow many of us to continue these attempts at establishing greater emotional intimacy with other men.

For some men, learning to extend the boundaries of friendship in new directions has not only become a fresh way to know themselves but also the opening of a new universe of experiences in emotional intimacy. However, this virgin territory already appears to be a mixed bag of positive and negative elements.

In respect to negative outcomes, some men have vocalized their having been hurt in terms of: (a) being openly rejected by one who was formerly their friend, (b) being open to negative labeling by friends and others who either misunderstand one's motivations or are threatened by them, (c) being susceptible to easy manipulation by those one has attempted to trust and with whom one has risked some deeper interaction, and (d) having to define themselves as persons who are dependent to some degree upon other men for emotional support.

The positive outcomes of initiating intimacy with other men have been described to us in terms of: (a) discovering new parts of the personality through learning to share and care for other males, (b) opening oneself to a novel range of previously unknown feelings and experiences, and (c) the growth of very satisfying and meaningful relationships with other men.

As one male participant evaluated his workshop experiences: "It's a shame that all my life I've been taught that I could love only one half of the human race, the female half. I'm really grateful that I'm now free of that limitation on my life."

REFERENCE NOTES

1. Pleck, J. *Male sex role behaviors in a representative national sample.* Paper presented at the Conference on New Research on Women, University of Michigan, 1975.
2. Verser, J. *Men and competition.* Unpublished manuscript, 1976.
3. Morin, S., & Wallace, S. *Traditional values, sex-role sterotyping and attitudes toward homosexuality.* Paper presented at the meeting of the Western Psychological Association, Los Angeles, April 1976.

4. Morin, S., Taylor, K., & Kielman, S. *Gay is beautiful at a distance.* Paper presented at the meeting of the American Psychological Association, Chicago, August, 1975.

REFERENCES

Argyle, M. *The psychology of interpersonal behavior.* Baltimore: Penguin, 1967.
Aries, E. Male/female interpersonal styles in all-male, all-female, and mixed groups. In A. G. Sargent (Ed.), *Beyond sex roles.* St. Paul: West & Co., 1976.
Balswick, J., & Peek, C. The inexpressive male: A tragedy of American society. *The Family Coordinator,* 1971, *20,* 363–368.
Bardwick, J., & Douvan, E. Ambivalence: The socialization of women. In V. Gornick & B. Moran (Eds.), *Women in sexist society.* New York: American Library, 1971.
Bem, S., Martyna, W., & Watson, C. Sex typing and androgyny: Further explorations of the expressive domain. *Journal of Personality and Social Psychology,* 1976, 334, 1016–1023.
Berkeley Men's Center. Berkeley Men's Center Manifesto. In J. H. Pleck & J. Sawyer (Eds.), *Men and masculinity,* Englewood Cliffs, N. J.: Prentice-Hall, 1974.
Brannon, R. The male sex role: Our culture's blueprint of manhood, and what it's done for us lately. In D. David & R. Brannon (Eds.), *The forty-nine percent majority: The male sex role.* Reading, Mass.: Addison-Wesley, 1976.
Chafetz, J. *Masculine/feminine, or human.* Itasca, Ill.: F. E. Peacock, 1974.
Clark, D. Homosexual encounter in all-male groups. In L. Solomon & B. Berzon (Eds.), *New perspectives on encounter groups.* San Francisco: Jossey-Bass, 1972.
DeGolia, R. Thoughts on men's oppression. *Issues in Radical Therapy,* 1973, 14–17.
Dickey, J. *Deliverance.* New York: Dell, 1970.
Fasteau, M. F. Why aren't we talking? *MS.,* 1972, *1*(1), 16.
Fasteau, M. F. *The male machine.* New York: McGraw-Hill, 1974.
Goldberg, H. *The hazards of being male: Surviving the myth of masculine privilege.* New York: Nash, 1976.
Harford, T. C., Willis, C. H., & Deabler, H. L. Personality correlates of masculinity-femininity. *Psychological Reports,* 1967, *21*(3), 881–884.
Hartley, R. Sex-role pressures in the socialization of the male child. *Psychological Reports,* 1959, *5,* 457–468.
Jourard, S. *The transparent self.* New York: D. Van Nostrand, 1971.
Jourard, S., & Landsman, M. J. Cognition, cathexis, and the "dyadic effect" in men's self-disclosing behavior. *Merrill-Palmer Quarterly,* 1960, *6,* 178–186.
Jourard, S., & Lasakow, P. Some factors in self-disclosure. *Journal of Abnormal and Social Psychology,* 1958, *56,* 91–98.
Jourard, S., & Richman, P. Factors in the self-disclosure inputs of college students. *Merrill-Palmer Quarterly,* 1963, *9,*141–148.
Kirkwood, J. *P.S. your cat is dead.* New York: Warner Communications, 1973.

Komarovsky, M. Patterns of self-disclosure of male undergraduates. *Journal of Marriage and the Family*, 1974, *36*, 677–686.

Komarovsky, M. *Dilemmas of masculinity: A study of college youth*. New York: Norton, 1976.

Knupfer, G., Clark, W., & Room, R. The mental health of the unmarried. *American Journal of Psychiatry*, 1966, *122*, 841–851.

Morin, S., & Garfinkle, E. M. Male homophobia. *Journal of Social Issues*, 1978, *34* (1), 29–47.

Mussen, P. Long-term consequents of masculinity of interests in adolescence. *Journal of Consulting Psychology*, 1962, *26*, 435–440.

Nye, F. I. *Role structure and analysis of the family*. Beverly Hills, Calif.: Sage, 1976.

Olstad, K. Brave new men: A basis for discussion. In J. Petras (Ed.), *Sex: Male/gender: Masculine*. Port Washington, New York: Alfred, 1975.

Pleck, J. My male sex role—and ours. *Win,* 1974, *10*, 8–12.

Pleck, J. Male-male friendship: Is brotherhood possible? In M. Glazer (Ed.), *Old family/new family: interpersonal relationships*. New York: Van Nostrand Reinhold, 1975. (a)

Pleck, J. Issues for the men's movement: Summer, 1975. *Changing Men: A Newsletter for Men Against Sexism*, 1975, 21–23. (b)

Pleck J., & Sawyer, J. (Eds.). *Men and masculinity*. Englewood Cliffs, N.J.: Prentice-Hall, 1974.

Powers, E., & Bultena, G. Sex differences in intimate friendships of old age. *Journal of Marriage and the Family*, 1976, *38*, 739–747.

Steinmann, A., & Fox, D. *The male dilemma*. New York: Jason Aronson, 1974.

Storey, D. *Radcliffe*, New York: Avon, 1963.

Szal, J. *Sex differences in the cooperative and competitive behaviors of nursery school children*. Unpublished master's thesis, Stanford University, 1972.

Vinacke, W. E. Sex roles in a three-person game. *Sociometry*, 1959. *22*, 343–360.

Vinacke, W. E., & Gullickson, G. R. Age and sex differences in the formation of coalitions. *Child Development*, 1964, *35*, 1217–1231.

Warren, P. N. *The front runner*. New York: Bantam Books, 1974.

Wolfgang, A., & Wolfgang, J. Exploration of attitudes via physical interpersonal distance toward the obese, drug users, homosexuals, police, and other marginal figures. *Journal of Clinical Psychology*, 1971, *27*, 510–512.

Males
In Psychotherapy

JERRY E. TOOMER
Dow Chemical USA
Midland, Michigan

Most men point to their head when asked to locate themselves imaginatively, and most women point to their chests [Nichols, 1975].

Theories of personality and psychotherapy along with psychological research have aroused the interest of mental health professionals and stimulated a great deal of debate regarding the negative effects of sex-role expectations on clients. However, little attention has been paid directly to effects of expectancy specifically on male clients, the issues that surround their treatment by both male and female therapists, and male clients' attitudes toward treatment. The thesis of this paper is that psychological treatment of all types should free men (and women) to incorporate optimal ways of thinking and feeling that result in flexible ways of behaving. In the discussion that follows I will examine background factors that have shaped our attitudes toward men, review research related to men in counseling and psychotherapy, and discuss implications for treatment.

The expectations of environment and the impact of powerful models and societal reinforcement, including mental health professionals, often contribute significantly to the shaping of life styles and goals of males. The impact of the environment is potentially so powerful that Stoller (1973) noted that biological predispositions determined by gender can be transcended; that is, personality traits of masculinity and femininity can be established by psychological influences such as reinforcement and modeling in opposition to biological male and female states.

The Six-Million-Dollar Man, Exo-Man, Firing Line, the Lombardian ethic, the Olympic Committee, to name a few, exhort young men to be super-males who are ingenious, competitive, physically powerful, and, most of all, winners. One of the Green Bay Packers' well-known players emerged from a superbowl victory saying, "We went out and won the game and preserved our manhood" (Nichols, 1975, p. 103). Although there has been no clear cause-effect relationship established between societal pressures and psychological reactions, examples of the possible effects of these expectations abound in our environment. Reputable studies conducted in the United States (Nichols, 1975) indicate that for every older woman who suicides there are seven older men who do the same. Apart from males' tendency to use more lethal means of self-injury, it would also appear that lack of communication of feelings, loneliness, isolation, and a resulting inability to elicit sympathetic responses from others may be contributing factors to this disproportionate suicide rate. Slaps on the back in shower rooms and on athletic fields are meager substitutes for meaningful human contact at a deeper level. Sheehy (1974) noted that only 5% of men over age 40 are unmarried, and that widowed or divorced men remarry sooner than widowed or divorced women. She offers the hypothesis that men are not emotionally equipped to live alone as well as women. Gorin, Veroff, and Feld (1960) indicated that unmarried men suffer far more from neurotic and antisocial tendencies and are often more depressed and passive than women who are unmarried. It appears to be the old bachelor, not the old maid, who suffers most from psychological distress. Valliant and McArthur (1972) noted that unmarried males tend to live out their lives like "latency boys," remaining bound to their mothers, underperforming in their careers, and spending little, if any, time living with a spouse. Further, Jourard's (1971) investigations of self-disclosure conclude that men keep their selves to themselves and impose an added burden of stress in addition to that imposed by everyday life. Their striving for a "manly" self-image becomes a kind of work whose chronic stress and energy expenditure may be a factor related to men's relatively shorter life-span. Some preliminary correlational data support the importance of stress as a contributor to decreased longevity. Friedman and Rosenman (1974) surveyed businessmen in the San Francisco area asking them to check what particular phenomenon or complex of habits they believed had preceded a heart attack in a friend of theirs. More than 70% believed that excessive competitive drive and meeting deadlines were the outstanding characteristics of their coronary-stricken friend. These characteristics, concomitant with a chronic sense of time urgency, form the basis of the Type A behavior pattern, which occurs so frequently among businessmen.

Horney (1974) proposed that even the "winners" (author's quotes) in American life feel insecure because they are aware of the mix of admiration and hostility directed at them. Colleagues wait for the chance to expose weakness; the faster gun challenges the proven gunfighter. Men in organizations are often reinforced for exciting and intellectual work that allows and encourages them to remain detached (Maccoby, 1976).

Preparation for becoming a "winner" often begins at an early age with career questions: Am I smart enough? Is my personality correct? Can I make "enough" money? And when they reach the point of having a relatively stable, secure career they become afraid that events beyond their control or their inability to control themselves will damage their success.

In summary, extensive evidence exists to support the contentions that a male sex-role stereotype operates to shape—and restrict—the values and actions of males in our society. Further, males appear to pay a price for conforming to a traditional masculine image as they die earlier, frequently live in self-imposed isolation, and suffer from an inordinate amount of stress. What are the implications for males in therapy? The following review will focus on client and therapist variables as they impact on men in treatment.

CLIENT VARIABLES

Several studies have investigated the expectations of clients prior to therapy, their reactions to therapy and therapists, and the duration and satisfaction with treatment. Tinsley and Harris (1976) reported that males expect counselors to be more directive, critical, and analytical while females expect more accepting and nonjudgmental counselors. Boulware and Holmes (1970) investigated university student preferences for potential therapists whose faces they viewed on slides. Both men and women preferred male therapists, however, when analyzed by problem type (educational-vocational or personal); male therapists were preferred for authoritative advice (educational-vocational concerns) while students preferred female therapists for understanding personal problems.

Clayton and Jellison (1975) found that males and females over a broad age range (adolescent through older adults) preferred male advisors. In a 1964 study, Fuller concluded that in general, most counseling center clients prefer male counselors prior to treatment presumably because of expectations of authority and prestige. It appears that, in general, clients select male therapists more often and for reasons of perceived authority and/or expertise, while some clients prefer female therapists for relating personal concerns.

Fuller (1963) investigated effects of sex of therapist on client behaviors during the counseling process. Results from a sample of educational-vocational clients indicated that males expressed less feeling during the interviews than females. There were no significant differences due to counselor sex; however, client/counselor dyads with at least one female were more likely to result in significantly more client self-disclosure than all-male dyads. Brooks (1974) supported Fuller's (1963) conclusions in finding that male client/counselor dyads resulted in less self-disclosure than dyads containing a female counselor or client. Similarly, Granthon (1973) examined initial interviews with Black students and found that clients explored themselves to a greater extent when a female rather than male counselor, White or Black, was present. In addition, Granthon noted that sex of therapist was a more significant variable in encouraging self-experience than was racial similarity.

Hill (1975) examined the effects of counselor experience level as it interacted with sex. She found that all-male or mixed-sex dyads were found to result in less discussion of feelings than all-female dyads and, further, that clients of both sexes reported more satisfaction with female therapists following the second interview. As noted in the above studies, it appears that male clients tend to disclose less, at least "early" in treatment, with male or female therapists, and that male client/male therapist dyads may be especially lacking in expression of feeling.

THERAPIST VARIABLES

Research pertaining to mental health professionals' judgments concerning the mental health of males and females is most aptly illustrated by the benchmark study of I. K. Broverman, D. M. Broverman, Clarkson, Rosenkrantz, and Vogel (1970). The authors concluded that clinicians held standards of mental health for men and women that paralleled the sex role stereotypes in our society. Much has been written about the adverse affect of this double standard on female clients, but what do research studies conclude regarding the impact of therapists' attitudes toward male clients? Broverman et al. noted that males were perceived as lacking interpersonal sensitivity, warmth, and expressiveness in comparison to females. More specifically, Haan and Livson (1973) investigated the sex differences of clinically experienced Ph.D.-level psychologists in the assessment of adult personalities. In comparison to female psychologist judges, males were generally more unfavorable in their assessments of both males and females. The authors speculated that male judges were especially reactive to "unmasculine" characteristics in men such as passivity and dependency. Additional support for the hypothesis that males have less favorable views of treatment and are less optimistic is given by Zeldow (1975). The author found that male students with a psychology background recommended psychiatric intervention significantly less often than females and were less optimistic than females regarding prognosis. Thomas and Stewart (1971) studied the responses of male and female counselors to audiotapes of five high school students with deviant and conforming career goals. The authors found that male counselors were less accepting of both deviate and conforming career goals than were female counselors.

Tanney and Birk (1976) concluded in a review of sex bias in counseling that most studies reported bias towards women on the part of both male and female counselors. It seems from the above review of the literature that a similar bias exists toward male clients.

MATCHING STUDIES

Several other studies have examined the effects of same and opposite sex matching. Persons (1973) researched therapists' characteristics and clients' improvement as perceived by clients at termination. The author found that even though all clients showed improvement as a result of psychotherapy, male clients were more responsive to male therapists and female clients more responsive to female therapists.

Daane and Schmidt (1957) found that both male and female counselors were rated higher on empathy when counseling clients of the same sex, indicating that counselors behave differently toward male and female clients in the interview. In a study of improvement rates, Cartwright and Lerner (1963) concluded that therapists had significantly higher empathy scores with patients of the opposite sex than with those of the same sex. However, the differences disappeared by the end of therapy and no difference in improvement rate was found.

Oleshan and Balter (1972) conducted a study investigating sex pairing and empathy with undergraduate students. They concluded that effectiveness was enhanced when a client had a counselor of the same rather than the opposite sex.

Mendelsohn (1966) studied the effects of client/counselor similarity on the duration of counseling. Although no significant differences were found, the author found that a higher proportion of continuers (91%) than terminators (46%) in the study were paired with a counselor of the same sex. In another study, Mendelsohn and Geller (1963) concluded that sex matching had little or no effect on length of counseling but that compatibility with therapist was related to outcome for female, but not male clients.

CONCLUSIONS FROM RESEARCH

What conclusions can be drawn from the research on client and therapist variables as they impact on males? Studies examining the presence and effects of sex bias in counseling are becoming more sophisticated as they incorporate additional variables such as race, client problem-type, duration of bias in treatment, and therapist age, theoretical orientation, and experience. Research is focusing less on sex bias per se and more on Bergin and Garfield's (1971) recommendation that psychologists clarify "what treatment for which client . . . under which circumstances." It is important to note that sex of therapist and client is only one variable.

Many investigations of sex bias and matching do seem to support the contention that sex role expectations by therapists do exist, expecially early in treatment as clients have stereotyped expectations and therapists react to demographic rather than personality characteristics of the client. Although mental health professionals tended to rate males more positively than females, it was also indicated that traditional male behavior is often expected of male clients, especially by male therapists. The "positive" view of male mental health may exact a price in that male clients are being encouraged to remain goal-oriented, relatively unfeeling, independent, and so forth.

There are a wide variety of possible reasons for the different treatment approaches or perceptions of male versus female clients. For example, Fabrikant (1974) reported that female patients were in therapy more than twice as long as male patients.

Do these data speak to the greater severity of concerns of female patients, to the ability of males to benefit from therapy in a shorter amount of time, to the bias of therapists in inaccurately perceiving females as less healthy, and keeping them in treatment, to the fear of male clients of remaining in treatment and exploring feelings, or to the bias of therapists in inaccurately viewing males as healthier and subsequently encouraging (or allowing) males to terminate prematurely?

In a report by the American Psychological Association Task Force on Sex Bias and Sex-Role Stereotyping in Psychotherapeutic Practice (1975) the results of an open-ended questionnaire indicated that women and children were preferentially referred or assigned to female therapists and men were referred to male therapists. The Task Force suggested that, as a minimum, therapists should be aware of their values and not impose them on the patient. Is this tendency to differentially assign male and female patients noted by the APA Task Force (1975) based on sound clinical judgment or is it the product of sex-bias among mental health professionals?

Researchers and therapists must work to clarify the above issues as they continue to sensitize themselves to the special needs and expectations of male patients. The author concurs with Tanney and Birk (1976) that it is difficult if not impossible at this point to clearly describe the effects of therapist and client sex on the process and outcome of treatment. Researchers must continue to clarify these issues by conducting more sophisticated investigations of sex effects per se, and by the control for and/or analysis of sex effects in psychotherapy research that will lead to more effective treatments for consumers of mental health services.

CONCLUSIONS AND IMPLICATIONS

Carter (1971) noted that much of male therapists' time in graduate training is spent in unlearning habits of emotional distance and restraint. She went on to suggest that multiple therapy teams should work to provide both cognitive (male therapist) and expressive (female therapist) models for the client. This approach, however, could serve to perpetuate the stereotypic behavior of therapists; the male therapist is brought in to fill the cognitive/reality testing role and is seen as not fully capable of providing an expressive model. Chesler (1971) hypothesized that all-male dyads encourage aggression and competition. Can male therapists, then, be the "good mother"—the accepting, supportive figure who skillfully encourages the male client to allow himself to become emotionally vulnerable in the therapy relationship (and other relationships as well) and, consequently, fully alive?

Male clients often enter treatment with expectations of male therapists as experts who will help them polish competitive skills and defenses. Also the pressure on the male therapist to "perform" early in treatment is often triggered by authority-expecting clients. Therapists must be especially aware of how they may explicitly or subtly encourage competition with male clients in the therapy relationship or encourage them to become even more controlling and emotionally stifled (obessive) in dealing with their environment.[1] If male therapy dyads have a notable lack of expression of feeling in treatment that restricts self-disclosure and exploration, therapists must evaluate their own biases and comfort—or discomfort—with expression of feeling. How do we react to statements of hopelessness, or extreme passivity, or a flow of tears from male clients? And how much more subjective stress must males experience before they can admit to the need for therapy, or once in therapy, share feelings of vulnerability with another male?

Theoretically, if the girl, according to psychoanalytic theory, is concerned that she once possessed a penis and lost it, the boy remains afraid of losing his (penis). The girl can "grieve," take stock of her unique strengths and go about living her life; the boy, however, continues to protect himself from feared loss of that beloved part (and the manliness it represents). If girls were hypothesized to be envious, boys must certainly be anxious. Anxious not only that they may lose their penis, but also anxious that someone may discover that its presence does not insure their power and competence; that they feel, after all, inferior even though they *have* a penis. They must, therefore, defend against the dreaded possibility that anyone, especially another male, discover their well-kept secret. Further, males' envy of woman's ability to give birth, provide nourishment through their breasts and "mother" is more successfully sublimated than the penis envy of the girl (Horney, 1974). Men, then, may overcompensate for their perceived small contribution to the creation of living beings by achieving in work and forms of play.

It may be that in long-term therapy the sex of therapists merely stimulates the patients to discuss their conflicts in a particular order. And, in the give and take of good psychotherapy, both becoming flexibly adaptable to society's expectations and acknowledging vulnerability and longings for nurturance are addressed. If the male therapist represents the father figure or male authority in the transference, many of the client's feelings may be those of competition, fearfulness, or perhaps deference to the "expert" in the extreme. We must ask ourselves who we are to this particular client at this particular time in the relationship, and further,

---

[1]This is not to say that *all* clients do not need and request assistance in becoming better able to stand up for their own rights and appropriately defend themselves. The goals of therapy are not to make males more passive or nonassertive, but rather to free them from the drive to be all-powerful, always in control, aggressive, etc.

decide how we can best respond to foster client growth. Certainly the impact of therapists, both male and female, as role models who can allow and encourage clients to explore themselves must be a crucial element of what we consider "good psychotherapy"—psychotherapy for better, not worse.

REFERENCES

American Psychological Association. Report of the task force on sex bias and sex role stereotyping in psychotherapeutic practice. *American Psychologist,* 1975, *30,* 1169–1175.

Bergin, A. E., & Garfield, S. L. *Handbook of psychotherapy and behavior change: An empirical analysis.* New York: Wiley, 1971.

Boulware, D., & Holmes, D. Preferences for therapists and related experiences. *Journal of Consulting and Clinical Psychology,* 1970, *35,* 269–277.

Brooks, L. Interactive effects of sex and status on self-disclosure. *Journal of Counseling Psychology,* 1974, *21,* 469–474.

Broverman, I. K., Broverman, D. M., Clarkson, F. E., Rosenkrantz, P., & Vogel, S. R. Sex-role stereotypes and clinical judgments of mental health. *Journal of Counseling and Clinical Psychology,* 1970, *34,* 1–7.

Carter, C. A. Advantages of being a woman therapist. *Psychotherapy: Theory, Research, and Practice,* 1971, *8,* 297–300.

Cartwright, R. D., & Lerner, B. Empathy, need to change, and improvement with psychotherapy. *Journal of Consulting Psychology,* 1963, *27,* 138–144.

Chesler, P. Patient and patriarch: Women in the psychotherapeutic relationship. In V. Gornick & B. Moran (Eds), *Women in sexist society: Studies in power and powerlessness.* New York: Basic Books, 1971.

Clayton, V., & Jellison, J. M. Preferences for the age and sex of advisors: A life span approach. *Developmental Psychology,* 1975, *11,* 861–862.

Daane, C., & Schmidt, L. G. Empathy and personality variables. *Journal of Educational Research,* 1957, *51,* 129–135.

Fabrikant, B. The psychotherapist and the female patient: Perceptions, misconceptions, and change. In V. Franks & V. Burtle (Eds.), *Women in therapy.* New York: Brunner/Mazel, 1974.

Friedman, M., & Rosenman, R. H. *Type A behavior and your heart.* New York: Knopf, 1974.

Fuller, F. Influence of sex of counselor and of client on client expression of feeling. *Journal of Counseling Psychology,* 1963, *10,* 34–40.

Fuller, F. Preferences for male and female counselors. *Personnel and Guidance Journal,* 1964, *42,* 463–467.

Gorin, G., Veroff, J., & Feld, S. *Americans view their mental helath.* New York: Basic Books, 1960.

Granthon, R. Effects of counselors sex, race, and language style on Black students in initial interviews. *Journal of Counseling Psychology,* 1973, *20,* 553–559.

Haan, N., & Livson, N. Sex differences in the eyes of expert personality assessors: Blind spots. *Journal of Personality Assessment,* 1973, *37,* 486–492.

Hill, C. E. Sex of client and sex and experience level of counselor. *Journal of Counseling Psychology,* 1975, *22,* 6–11.

Horney, K. The flight from womanhood: The masculinity complex in women as viewed by men and by women. In J. Strouse (Ed.), *Women and analysis*. New York: Grossman, 1974.

Jourad, S. *The transparent self*. New York: Van Nostrand, 1971.

Maccoby, M. *The gamesman: The new corporate leaders*. New York: Simon & Schuster, 1976.

Mendelsohn, G. A. Effects of client personality and client/counselor similarity on the duration of counseling: A replication and extension. *Journal of Counseling Psychology*, 1966, *13*, 228–234.

Mendelsohn, G. A., & Geller, M. H. Effects of counselor/client similarity on the outcome of counseling. *Journal of Counseling Psychology*, 1963, *10*, 71–77.

Nichols, J. *Men's liberation: A new definition of masculinity*. New York: Penguin Books, 1975.

Oleshan, W., & Balter, L. Sex and empathy. *Journal of Counseling Psychology*, 1972, *19*, 559–562.

Persons, W. E. Occupational prediction as a function of the counselor's racial and sexual bias. (Doctoral dissertation, University of Florida, 1972.) *Dissertation Abstracts International*, 1973, *34*, 139A–140A. (University Microfilms, No. 73–15, 533.)

Sheehy, G. *Passages: Predictable crises of adult life*. New York: Dulton, 1974.

Stoller, R. J. The "bedrock" of masculinity and femininity: Bisexuality. In J. Miller (Ed.), *Psychoanalysis and women*. Baltimore: Penguin Books, 1973.

Tanney, M. F., & Birk, J. M. Women counselors for women clients? A review of the research. *The Counseling Psychologist*, 1976, *6*(2), 28–32.

Thomas, A., & Stewart, N. Counselor response to female clients with deviate and conforming career goals. *Journal of Counseling Psychology*, 1971, *18*, 352–357.

Tinsley, H. E., & Harris, D. J. Client expectations for counseling. *Journal of Counseling Psychology*, 1976, *23*, 173–177.

Valliant, G., & McArthur, C. Natural history of male psychologic health: The adult life cycle from 18–50. *Seminar in Psychiatry*, November 1972, *4*.

Zeldow, P. B. Clinical judgment: A search for sex differences. *Psychological Reports*, 1975, *37*, 1135–1142.

Holland's Typology Applied to Client/Counselor Interaction: Implications for Counseling with Men

MONROE A. BRUCH

Bradley University*

"Why do many men not seek counseling or experience dissatisfaction and failure in counseling?" is a question asked frequently by counselors. It is an accepted fact that more women than men seek counseling regardless of setting or type of service. Popular reasons given for this situation are that: (a) women are more prone to emotional difficulties due to their role and status in society and (b) men tend to view the seeking of help as contrary to their sex role expectations. While these conclusions are intuitively reasonable, they remain largely untested due to a lack of systematic theorizing and data collection. Bergin and Garfield's (1971) broad coverage of psychotherapy research contains, for example, little mention of client sex and willingness to seek services or client sex and progress in therapy.

Clinical experience provides another reminder of the continuing difficulties with male clients. For example, my experience with one male client seems representative of some of the common issues encountered when working with men. Ray is a 39-year-old technical worker whom I was counseling with respect to his marital problems and his feelings of anxiety. Ray was reluctant to come to sessions and attended only upon his wife's insistence. Despite my empathic responding to his reluctance toward counseling, Ray demonstrated little self-disclosure of feelings. In later sessions he questioned the value of "just talking" and wanted me to tell him something to do to make things better at home. In joint sessions, I attempted to improve marital interaction by use of communication, conflict resolution, and social contracting skills all of which the wife learned and

It is important for a clear understanding and critical examination of the ideas presented in this article that readers be familiar with Holland's theory (Holland, 1973). The author assumes responsibility for his approach to generalizing Holland's typology to client/counselor interaction, and the viewpoints expressed should not be misconstrued as representative of Holland's original theory or intentions. Appreciation is expressed to Harold Benner and the editors for their constructive feedback on the article.
*Now at State University of New York at Albany.

practiced but Ray did not. Thereafter, I tried working with him individually using our relationship, even sharing my feelings of anger, to process communication difficulties. There was, however, little therapeutic gain.

Not wanting to admit my helplessness, I fantasized various solutions to our dilemma. Again and again, however, my thoughts returned to an analysis of our social interaction. As a counselor, I believed Ray needed to improve communication skills with his spouse and children, to disclose feelings about his father's death, to deal with problems relating to sexual functioning, and to value other interpersonal matters. However, Ray's skills and interests lay in mechanical activities. He preferred discussing motorcycles as opposed to interpersonal matters and viewed his role at home as taking responsibility for material and financial affairs.

Thus, it seemed that Ray, like other men with whom I worked, did not fit into the counseling process the way it is usually practiced. The counseling environment, like any other environment, demands a unique set of skills, competencies, interests, and values from the client. Within the counseling environment, the client is reinforced for exhibiting skills of self-expression—for example; verbal, assertive, self-disclosing, and insightful—and the client is rewarded for holding values of cooperativeness and seeing the importance of interpersonal over material concerns. In turn the counselor is also a person within an environment created by the client's behavior. In sessions with clients who lack skill and interest in self-expression and interpersonal matters, the counselor experiences less reward for his/her participation. Consequently, the current analysis provoked a question relevant to both Ray and many other male clients, "Could the issue of men in counseling be better understood as a problem of person/environment matching?" Specifically, if many male clients do not behave in ways that match the type of competencies and values rewarded by the traditional counseling environment, then an analysis of counseling as a problem in person/environment interaction may suggest some tentative solutions.

One model of person/environment interaction relevant to an analysis of client/counselor interaction is Holland's (1973) typology of persons and environments. In the remainder of this article, I will apply his typology to the client/counselor relationship for the purpose of suggesting potential reasons for failure and success with male clients. First, using the hexagonal model, expected effects on interaction resulting from the degree of congruence/incongruence of the six personality types with the social environment of counseling is explored. As a part of this process, additional Holland concepts of consistency and differentiation are integrated with congruence to extend the usefulness of the typology. Second, implications from the typology for previous counseling research on facilitative core conditions, client pretraining, and social psychological variables of attitude change are discussed. Third, implications of the typology for differential use of counseling techniques, goal-setting, and design of alternative counseling services are also elaborated. While the focus of this application is on male clients, Holland's theory is relatively sex role independent thus making the discussion relevant for female clients. Finally, my generalization of Holland's theory to social interaction in counseling is not intended to explain all aspects of interaction nor is the reader to draw conclusions concerning the relative potency of these variables as opposed to variables proposed by others. The scope of this article is exploratory and descriptive. The ideas presented are intended to generate future research that may provide a better understanding of how males may or may not respond to counseling.

HOLLAND'S TYPOLOGY APPLIED TO CLIENT-COUNSELOR INTERACTION

Holland's (1973) theory of career choice is also a theory about personality and social interaction. Because he assumes that vocational preference stems from personality and environmental determinants, his theory provides a useful method for assessing outcomes of both career choice and social behavior. While the latter emphasis is virtually unacknowledged and unresearched, it is implicit in Holland's (1973) writing. His research suggestions (Holland, 1973, p. 145) exhort the reader to investigate student/teacher, client/counselor, employee/supervisor, and husband/wife interactions using this system. Also, in a recent reexamination of the theory, Holland and Gottfredson (1976) extend the fundamental concepts of the model to adult development thereby using Holland's principles to explain some aspects of social behavior. The primary content of Holland's theory consists of the six basic personality types. These types are classed as Realistic (R), Investigative (I), Artistic (A), Social (S), Enterprising (E), and Conventional (C), along with their corresponding model environments. More important to this article are Holland's methods for analyzing information about person types and environments. The concepts of congruence, consistency, and differentiation are the basic tools of the system for hypothesizing differential outcomes for various person/environment pairings. Congruence is defined as the relationship between the individual's personality type and any of the six model environments based on the hexagonal model (Holland, 1973, p. 23). High congruence is illustrated by an S type individual in group counseling (S environment) as compared to an S type working on a bookkeeping task (C environment). Consistency refers to the degree of integration among the various skills and values within a person's behavior pattern or within an environment (that is, another individual or group of people) based again on the hexagon. In terms of social interaction, more predictable outcomes are expected when both person and environmental consistency are high—for example, SA type counselor leading Personal Growth Group (SA environment)—in contrast to situations where person consistency is high and environment consistency is low

Androgynous High masculine High feminine IAS, ISA, A, AIS, AIR	*Feminine* High Feminine Low Masculine S, SA, AS, SEA, ASE
Masculine High masculine R, RI, RC, RIE, RIC, IR	*Undifferentiated* Low Differentiation (for example, little difference between highest & lowest Holland code)

Figure 1. Classification of some Holland types according to predominant sex-role attributes

or where both are low. Differentiation is defined as the absolute raw score difference between a person's highest and lowest scores on the six personality scales of the Vocational Preference Inventory (VPI) (Holland, 1973). When both the person and environment are highly differentiated (for example, a 40-year-old machinist, R type, working with a RI type 55-year-old bench lathe operator) the satisfaction and productivity will be more predictable in contrast to a situation in which two college students (one undecided, the other considering majors in law or engineering) are working in similar factory positions. With Holland's three components for assessing person/environment interaction now defined, we proceed in applying the typology to client/counselor interaction.

Counseling as a social environment. Among the six types, S best describes not only the personality of the counselor but the traditional counseling process. Being an S environment, the counseling situation requires competencies and interests in verbal ability such as self-disclosure of thoughts and feelings, abstract thinking and problem-solving, and other interpersonal skills such as empathy, self-monitoring, and insight as to how others see one's behavior. In turn the environment (counselor) selectively rewards these abilities and values since they appear essential to the goals of behavioral change. Also, the more specialized the professional setting and sophisticated the counselor's training/experience the more likely the environment possesses higher degrees of differentiation and consistency. For instance, a Ph.D. psychologist with 7 years experience in a university psychological clinic is likely to represent an environment (for example, a counselor and a setting) with higher differentiation and consistency than a teacher of Business/Education courses working part time as a school counselor. The higher the consistency and differentiation of the service setting and counselor, the more intense the demand on the client to conform to the S environment. Conversely, when a wider spectrum of counseling services is considered, it is possible to find more varied counseling environments (ES or ASE types such as Job Corps, Admissions Counseling, and Drama Therapy) with lesser degrees of consistency and/or differentiation in those doing the counseling (for example, some paraprofessional counselors, administrators, or those in teaching/research roles).

While the usual counseling situation represents an S environment, the personality types of persons seeking counseling vary across the six Holland types. A majority of men appear to possess Holland codes of R, I, and E tending to place them at positions on the hexagon less correlated with the S environment of counseling. To the contrary, findings by Gottfredson and Holland (1975) tend to support the notion that many women appear to possess S or SA personality types. Thus, at its simplest level the typology suggests initially that males more than females may possess personality types less congruent with counseling. However, Holland's typology is helpful at this point because it does not restrict us to a simple dichotomy of maleness/femaleness. Both in psychology and in society at large, masculinity and femininity have long been conceptualized as bipolar ends of a single dimension. Recently scholars in a number of disciplines have focused on the concept of psychological androgyny, a term denoting the integration of both masculinity and femininity within a single individual (Bem, 1974; 1977). The concept implies that an individual can be both assertive and compassionate, or instrumental and expressive, all depending on the situational appropriateness of these responses. Scoring on this dimension is pictured via a fourfold table ranging from high scores on both masculinity and femininity dimensions to low on both signifying lack of differentiation. Holland's theory accommodates the concept of androgyny because the six types encompass a universe of related but distinct behavior styles, some containing both masculine and feminine orientations, while others contain more traits of one than the other. As illustrated in Figure 1 some Holland types can be categorized according to this fourfold table. This figure is intended as a heuristic device to clarify the fact that client/counselor congruence/incongruence is not solely a problem of sex role differences. According to the figure, males may possess various combinations of both masculine and feminine characteristics with R, RI, RC, and IR types possessing predominately male characteristics; A, S, and SA types more female orientations; and IAS types being more androgynous. Males and females with types reflecting androgyny or predominantly female characteristics are assumed more congruent with the demands of the counseling experience. Two obvious correlaries are that R, C, and IR female clients and clients of either sex with low differentiation possess characteristics less congruent with counseling.

Expected interaction outcomes with the six client types. In this section the advantages or disadvantages created by the particular behavior style of each type is delineated for client/counselor interaction. While this discussion is simplistic because most individuals are some combination of types, it provides some basic tenets when considering both single and more complex two or three code types. With the R type (recall Ray, my client discussed earlier), counselor communication (verbal stimuli) contains limited rewarding power other than creating the normal convivial atmosphere expected in a professional setting. Where the counselor assumes that responses ranging from reflection of feelings to confrontation are rewarding because they convey acceptance or stimulate client awareness of contradictory behavior, the R type individual possesses a different reinforcement history making him less responsive to this form of influence. Also, the counseling procedures used to remediate typical concerns brought to counseling—such as marital discord, social anxiety, nonassertiveness, and other problem-solving difficulties—involve the very skills, information, philosophy, and values that the R type is lacking. Consequently, the counselor may experience little satisfaction when working with this type because many interpersonal skills are absent and progress may be inconsistent.

Similar to the R personality, the C type client's proclivity for manipulation of data and organization of material things predisposes this person to avoid less structured interpersonal and exploratory activities such as counseling. This type may be uneasy in expressing personal feelings, unimaginative and inhibited in interpersonal problem-solving. Such individuals may expect counseling to be a highly structured and impersonal procedure. Also, this client's need to conform and to follow traditional social roles may prevent seeking of counseling and/or may create an unwillingness to participate in certain counseling activities. For example, the liberal attitudes and unstructured nature of some humanistic counseling approaches like Gestalt techniques may be perceived as aversive. The C types' behavior may be nonrewarding to the counselor as well because the counselor is approached as an authority on the presenting problem from whom expert answers and solutions are expected. Counselors are likely to perceive clients with predominately C and R orientations as "defensive" because they manifest a question/answer style of interaction without a willingness for personal disclosure.

In contrast, A, E, and I types evidence a mixture of facilitating and inhibiting predispositions that places them at an intermediate level of congruence to the S type counselor. With the A type, there are competencies and interests in self-expression leading to exploration of personal feelings and more satisfaction from unstructured, introspective counseling procedures. However, the concomitant impulsive and emotive style of the A type may also mean the client is unable to organize his/her report of feelings or maintain focus on particular feelings. Any structure imposed by the environment may be resented, and ground rules for taking responsibility may be tested by the A type. Rewards to the counselor may be limited by this client's tendency to be vague, idealistic, and complicated. Flitting from topic to topic or use of manipulative tactics such as verbal games of ''I don't know'' or ''Yes, but . . . '' may frustrate systematic progress. Clinical experience suggests that often A types are the "groupies" or clients that go from counselor to counselor never being quite satisfied. Similar to the A type, the developmental history of the E personality predisposes him/her not only toward verbal skills, but also manipulation and verbal aggression in social interaction. The desire to be "correct" and sell one's point of view may limit the client's capacity to listen to counselor feedback. Thus, genuine self-exploration and "owning" individual responsibility for problems may be superficial. Psychological techniques discussed as a genuine means of improving social relationships may be inadvertently used for controlling others. Disconcerting to the counselor is the observation that the E type can speak the language of self-improvement but not necessarily live it.

To the contrary, the I type potentially brings skills and interests in intellectual awareness to the problem-solving task of traditional counseling. The I type is an astute processor potentially showing quick insight following counselor feedback. However, this client may devalue the importance of feelings and perhaps limit progress in behavior change. The I type's choosing to remain "in their computer" may frustrate a counselor's expectations for exploration of feelings. Tendencies to be highly critical both of self and counselor may manifest itself in obsessive questioning or resistance to trying different behavior change strategies. With I types, secondary personality characteristics take on added importance. Depending on whether the secondary features are toward the R or AS personality type may increase or decrease the degree of congruence.

Potentially the S type possesses those competencies, perceptions, and attitudes most congruent with counseling. Self-referral rather than referral by others is probably higher for this individual. Preference for educational, self-development, and interpersonal activities may make such individuals responsive to a wider range of counseling techniques than are other types. Their learning history not only makes them responsive to counselor communication modes but in turn they may reciprocate empathy toward the counselor. While clients with SA codes will find counseling highly rewarding and respond more consistently, S types with nonadjacent or opposite secondary characteristics (SC, SR) may evidence less consistent responsiveness.

The preceding section discussed effects arising primarily from degrees of client congruence/incongruence with the counseling environment. Assessing the counseling relationship in terms of congruence plus consistency and differentiation of both client and environment, however, extends the practical application of Holland's theory. Interactions based on different degrees of congruence, consistency, and differentiation greatly increase the range of situations evaluated by the typology. Three case illustrations of low, moderate, and high client-to-counselor congruence in combination with varying degrees of client consistency and differentiation are presented to demonstrate how differential outcomes result when these three methods are combined.

As depicted in Figure 2, because of the R type's low congruence with the counseling environment, higher or lower degrees of client consistency and differentiation have little effect in overcoming the problems created by initial incongruence. A highly differentiated and consistent RI person may be a 40-year-old, male mechanic while the RSE individual is perhaps a confused, dependent 20-year old with poorly developed goals. Although for different reasons, the personality patterns of all the clients represented in Figure 2 suggest that they would find counseling unattractive because it demands competencies, interests, and self-perceptions which they lack or which are in opposition to their reinforcement history.

The second case is an I type client representing an intermediate level of congruence. With congruence at this level, consistency of personality as measured by the individual's two- or three-point Holland code takes on a unique function in moderating predictions of outcomes. Specifically, high consistency is facilitative when the direction is toward an ISA or IAS orientation. When the direction is toward IR, however, high consistency magnifies problems resulting from incongruence. Therefore, high consistency is not uniformly beneficial with this type in contrast to high differentiation which increases behaviors indicative of the individuals's dominant personality type. These conclusions are illustrated in Figure 3 by comparing the variations in the upper and lower sections. It is assumed that the high consistency and differentiation of the IAS, ISA type enable the person to apply analytical and introspective skills to interpersonal matters. In the same context, the skills and values associated with the IR type

		Consistency	
	Low	Moderate	High
Differentiation Low	RSE	REA	RIS
Moderate	RS E	RE A	RI S
High	RS E	RE A	RI S

Figure 2. Examples of low client/counselor congruence (realistic personality of client) combined with varying degrees of consistency and differentiation. Size of letters denotes degree of consistency, and distance between third and first letters denotes differentiation.

| | Consistency | | |
	Low	Moderate	High
Differentiation			
Low	IES	ISE	IAE
Moderate	IE S	IS E	IA E
High	IE S	IS E	IA E
Low	IES	ICE	IRE
Moderate	IE S	IC E	IR E
High	IE S	IC E	IR E

Figure 3. Examples of intermediate client/counselor congruence (investigative personality of client) combined with varying levels of consistency and differentiation. Size of letter denotes degree of consistency, and distance between third and first letter denotes differentiation.

enable this person to be equally capable in analytical skills but to prefer to apply them to mechanical/technical tasks not interpersonal. The IAS, ISA type's competencies and interests increase the individual's awareness of self and other's actions and attitudes heightening responsiveness to counseling tasks.

When the client possesses high congruence, as with the S type individual, it is assumed that dimensions of consistency and differentiation interact in an either/or fashion. As demonstrated in Figure 4, when both

| | Consistency | | |
	Low	Moderate	High
Differentiation			
Low	SR	SIR	SAR
Moderate	S R	SI R	SA R
High	S R	SI R	SA R

Figure 4. Examples of high client/counselor congruence (social personality of client) combined with varying levels of consistency and differentiation. Size of letter denotes degree of consistency, and distance between third and first letter denotes differentiation.

factors are high the attitudes, motivation, and interpersonal skills brought to counseling afford a desirable match with the counselor's role behaviors. Perhaps degree of differentiation is slightly more important than consistency because when elevated there is less variability in the client's responsiveness to the counseling process which serves to make the interaction more rewarding for the counselor.

Research in Client/Counselor Interaction

In this section implications of Holland's typology are discussed in relation to previous findings in client/counselor interaction. While a variety of topics exist, I selected three areas that have received extensive attention in the counseling literature.

The first variable is Rogerian facilitative conditions. The importance of facilitative conditions of empathy, genuineness, and unconditional positive regard were proposed by Rogers (1957) and examined extensively by Truax and Carkhuff (1967), Carkhuff (1969), and Truax and Mitchell (1971). Purportedly high levels of therapist functioning on these response variables increased effectiveness of both counseling process and outcome variables. While the empirical support for separate distinctions among these constructs and their exact relationship to counseling outcome is highly equivocal (Gormally & Hill, 1974; Gladstein, 1977; Lambert & De Julio, 1977), results from some studies suggest that these variables may increase client self-disclosure of affect and subsequent feelings of self-esteem. Particularly relevant to our discussion of client/counselor interaction is additional evidence that client variability in disclosing personal feelings has a reciprocal impact on therapists' continued expression of facilitative responses (Carkhuff & Alexik, 1967; Friel, Dratochevil, & Carkhuff, 1968).

Examination of these findings from the perspective of Holland's typology suggests that certain qualifications be considered when making generalizations about the uniform nature and effects of facilitative core conditions in counselor training and client/counselor interaction. With respect to counselor training in empathy skills, the typology suggests that development of competencies and attitudes leading to higher levels of counselor response are a product of both training and personality orientation. Using Holland's model of personality development, differences in counselor level of response may be explained by varying degrees of congruence, consistency, and differentiation. For example, the ES type counselor may be more "business-like" in communication consequently showing greater variability and attaining only moderate levels on empathy ratings. However, the single code S type counselor with high differentiation may evidence consistently higher levels of facilitative response. The typology also implies that client self-exploration influences subsequent counselor empathy levels. The differentiated S type counselor may persist

In high levels of response because it is self-rewarding regardless of client responsiveness where less consistent and differentiated counselor personality types are affected by client unresponsiveness and switch to other modes of communication.

The notion that facilitative core conditions are always important for all clients is questioned by the typology. Perhaps these communication modes are "core conditions" for S, A, and some E types but not necessarily for R, C, and some I types. Thus counselor behaviors such as empathy do not obtain their potency or effectiveness over other communication approaches due to some inherent nature. Rather, any verbal response whether reflection or simple instruction acquires its potency through antecedent characteristics of the client personality type that predispose the person to particular verbal interpersonal modes.

A second area of investigation into client/counselor interaction is client preparation for psychotherapy or client pretraining. Gaining impetus from Schofield's (1964) analysis of contemporary psychotherapy and his resultant description of the YAVIS (young, attractive, verbal, intelligent, and successful) client who is highly preferred by therapists, techniques were developed such as role induction (Orne & Wender, 1968; Strupp & Bloxom, 1973) and vicarious pretraining (Truax, Shapiro, & Wargo, 1968). Such procedures were designed for the Non-YAVIS client (Goldstein, 1971) who is typically lower class, restricted in verbalization, nonempathic, oriented to material needs, and who externalizes concerns by defining problems as physical rather than stemming from personal irrationality. Goldstein (1973, pp. 1–52) presents an excellent discussion of the personality development of the lower-class client which describes the development of language styles and belief systems uncomplimentary to the typical counseling process. Many of the client attributes and language behaviors described by Goldstein are strikingly similar to Holland's definition of R, C, and some I types. Perhaps some of my conclusions, based on generalizations from Holland's model, could be predicted simply by considering the client's social class. Both lines of thinking, however, arrive at the same set of questions. Should we view lower-class (low congruence R, C, IR) clients as not ready for counseling, thereby striving to prepare them to talk our language? Or, should we acknowledge a general lack of effectiveness with this type client and instead develop different strategies of intervention?

Some tentative responses to these questions about client pretraining are suggested by the typology. First, client unsuitability is no longer viewed as a deficit in one or two traits like speech style or social skill but as an inherently different personality style that will endure after counseling is terminated. Thus, one can question the value or permanence of a "change" effected by teaching an R type male the communication skills and other interpersonal values of an S type orientation when one knows that he will return to an R environment—for example, factory job, mechanical activities, and R type spouse. Secondly, the typology suggests that pretraining may be preferred for client types more congruent with the S orientation (A, E, and IAS) while R, C, and IR types might benefit from alternative forms of intervention. In the former case pretraining via modeling, role-playing, instructions, and counselor reinforcement might capitalize on similar characteristics that E, A, and ISA types share with the S orientation and thereby increase responsiveness to the counseling process. Also, S types with lower differentiation and consistency may benefit from pretraining because of their initial similarity with the environment. On the other hand, R, C, and IR clients may show only superficial change following pretraining and should be offered treatment environments more congruent with their personality. Action-oriented services, educational programs, on-the-job training, paraprofessional services, and community psychology approaches may afford interventions that possess more characteristics in common with R, C, and IR orientations than traditional verbal psychotherapy.

A third topic area in client/counselor interaction stems from the extrapolation of findings from experimental social psychology research on attitude change, social power, and verbal conditioning (Goldstein & Simonson, 1971; Strong, 1968; Schmidt & Strong, 1970; Strong & Dixon, 1971; Strong & Matross, 1973). These authors and others have studied counselor influence in terms of counselor/client attraction, counselor expertness, status, trustworthiness, and counselor responding as differential reinforcement. In general, a majority of the variance for any of these factors arises from basic effects of social reinforcement. My application of Holland's typology has also been cast in terms of social reinforcement concepts. Consequently, the similarity between interpersonal attraction variables in client/counselor interaction and Holland's concept of congruence is obvious from my previous discussion and has been studied by Hogan, Hall, and Blank (1972). Less obvious is the value of the typology to make differential predictions about interpersonal influence variables. To date research has treated constructs such as similarity-attraction as unitary factors when arranging verbal or behavioral stimuli designed to enhance or diminish its effects. Unique characteristics of the six Holland types suggest varied responsiveness to the stimuli that constitute attractiveness, expertise, or trustworthiness. E and C types may be influenced more by conventional manipulation of stimuli conveying status, while A and I types may construe expertise or prestige differently or even find it aversive. In the case of R types, attractiveness and expertise are better enhanced by use of action-oriented counseling procedures rather than a verbal-intuitive process. Paraprofessionals possessing similar occupational-cultural backgrounds to R types may be rated more attractive and skilled than the typical professional. Attributes conveying trustworthiness may differ among types. For instance, S types are more sensitive to suggestions of breach of confidence or ulterior motives, while for other types presence or absence of these cues produce no predictable effects. Finally, the role of consistency and differentation could be to strengthen predictability of the effects from manipulations of attractiveness, expertise, and trustworthiness because the individual is less variable in responsiveness to those cues used to represent these factors.

Male Client's Personality Type and Selection of Counseling
Methods and Goals

In this final section, alternative approaches to the design and delivery of services to men suggested by the typology are examined. The discussion focuses on problems resulting from how males get into counseling, different counseling approaches depending on Holland personality type, and establishing counseling goals with regard to type.

Because of the particular skills, attitudes, and values of the S, SA, ES, ISA, and some A types, males with these orientations may perceive counseling as useful and nonthreatening and seek services before problems become incapacitating. To the contrary, males with R, C, and IR personalities hold incongruent skills and attitudes and may avoid counseling when problems arise. Thus, many R, C, and IR type males arrive at counseling by agency referral at a time when their problems may have reached crisis proportions. In a crisis the incongruencies created by their preference for action rather than introspection, expectations of receiving solutions, and other value differences are magnified. Such incongruities also affect follow through. That is, once the crisis is met, such clients do not return to the counseling setting since they conclude that their problems are solved. Thus, the earlier question about pretraining the incongruent client for the treatment environment versus changing the mode of intervention is compounded by the reality that many males arrive for counseling at a time when their suffering prevents them from taking personal responsibility for their concerns.

For R, C, and IR types professional counselors need to develop and provide improved access to alternative treatment programs. For example, a preventive or community psychology model may have advantages for less congruent R, C, and IR types because the structure of services can incorporate learning and behavior change approaches more compatible with their personality styles. Employing an adult education or continuing education format to deliver information and training experiences in assertive, marital, parenting, and behavioral self-control skills involves the male as a student rather than a client. For those who would self-select out of such programs, providing inservice education programs in these areas during working hours in business and industry may afford utilization of social modeling influences by co-workers who willingly attend, thus encouraging participation. Such alternatives allow the persons to receive assistance in their preferred environment.

Since interventions should approximate the values, expectations and other qualities of R, C, and IR environments, it may be important that those providing direct service possess personality style compatible with the client's. Consequently, the counselor acts as a consultant to other agencies having frequent contact with incongruent personality types. For example, training of police and other law enforcement personnel in family intervention and other interpersonal problem-solving methods may increase behavior change more effacaciously than one-to-one counseling.

While the typology suggests that we move toward nontraditional strategies for incongruent males, the general task remains to delineate particular behavior change methods best suited for each type. Advantages of certain counseling methods with specific types, anticipated client reactions to these methods and selection of counseling goals are elaborated below. The use of direct counseling approaches employing simple instructions, examples, and guided practice seems desirable for R, C, and IR type clients because of their preference for structured activities and action rather than symbolic-introspective activities. Various behavioral counseling approaches emphasizing modeling, instructions, guided practice, social contracts, and self-management might meet with more interest and commitment because their rationale and implementation is straightforward and more similar to traditional learning environments like the classroom or work station. The use of reading materials and "apparatus" such as programmed learning or computer assisted materials and self-operated audio or videotape materials may appeal to this client's desire for structure, manipulation of materials, and more impersonal approaches to problem-solving. Counselors in both clinical and educational settings report that some clients prefer working with such apparatus and materials rather than a counselor. Programs such as the System of Interactive Guidance Information (SIGI) (Katz, 1974) in vocational counseling and self-operated, automated treatment programs in community mental health settings (Elwood, 1975) are illustrations of approaches suited to individuals with these personality types. The use of structured behavioral procedures assumes the rationale of specific goal setting. Step-by-step goal setting seems especially valuable for less congruent types because it inhibits the imposition of S type values and attitudes on the client. This manner of goal setting may have far reaching implications to the extent that the behaviors, preferences, and attitudes of the R, C, and IR type client are viewed more positively by counselors since these personality characteristics are adaptive when the client returns to his R, C, IR social, educational, and work environment.

The ISA or IA type male's analytical approach to problem-solving suggests several strategies. In general, he may benefit from counselor presentation of why certain behaviors need to be altered and how selected procedures will accomplish the task. Cognitive-behavior therapy approaches including rational-emotive and behavioral self-control procedures seem highly relevant since they emphasize the individual as a personal scientist who is constantly hypothesizing about self and environment and modifying behavior accordingly. Also, these approaches deal with client feelings (effective behavior) in a manner more acceptable to the I's orientation than do some humanistic or phenomenological approaches. Again, counseling goals are delimited and the client is highly involved in determining his own goals.

Because A type clients tend to be expressive, intuitive, emotive, and liberal in their orientation, they prefer less conventional counseling approaches. Group counseling that emphasizes exercises from Gestalt, Transactional Analysis, Psychodrama, NTL and other consciousness-raising procedures contain opportunities for self-expressive behavior and peer interaction. This type of counseling atmosphere and method may decrease the A type's resistance to approach behavior change programs, channel profuse expressiveness toward self-change via group feedback, and reduce early termination because expressiveness is rewarded by the group. Such methods deemphasize clinical history taking, strict goal setting and attainment plus homework assignments while emphasizing the "here and now" and creative problem solving. Also, a variety of Humanistic and Ego Psychology approaches are oriented to the exploration of feelings and ambiguous verbal-symbolic processes which are compatible with the skills and interests of the A personality.

The unique characteristics of the E type predisposes this client to desire an active counselor role where the therapist uses rational, persuasive, and perhaps confrontive approaches to change client behavior. Counseling that employs a mixture of Rational-Emotive, Transactional Analysis, and Gestalt methods to expose "games" and attitudes stemming from hidden agendas may be more effective and meaningful to this client. The relatively exclusive emphasis on verbal manipulation of attitudes rather than the systematic observation, recording, and practice of alternative responses emphasized by behavioral approaches is perhaps preferred by the E male client. Also, the influence of counselor expertise and attractiveness on attitude change may assume a greater role with this Holland type. Challenges offered by social contracts such as earning back or forfeiting a money deposit as an inducement for change may prove fruitful if a tendency to manipulate or rationalize (both E type skills) can be avoided. Also, structured group tasks involving simulations via role-playing offer other ways of conveying therapeutic information. Counseling goals with the E type, like the A type, need repeated evaluation because of client desire for control of the relationship and superficiality in commitment to behavior change.

With the S type client, the therapeutic relationship takes on added importance regardless of whether a phenomological or behavioral approach is used. The S type is perhaps more adaptable than other types to a wider spectrum of counseling approaches provided that such approaches are couched in an emphatic interpersonal environment. A desire to cooperate and please the counselor increases the client's willingness to respond to various counseling procedures. However, an atmosphere in which the client can both give and receive seems valuable because of interests in others' welfare, self-development, and educational activities. Programs that involve the S type as a helper, peer counselor, or tutor provide a therapeutic function for this client. The act of being a helper leads to the kinds of reinforcements about one's importance and skills that are especially valued by the S type. Secondly, the response practice that results from a helper-therapy approach affords another influence on the client's behavior.

Counseling goals with the S, SA, or SE client will often include broader areas of functioning because of his desire for continued development of insight into self. Extended therapy may be more valuable for this type because personal growth and change is a major interest. Movement from individual to group programs or vice versa is a common clinical phenomenon with individuals possessing S orientations. More importantly fading of therapist-directed learning to self-management is facilitated by the skill and values characteristic of this type.

Like most writers, I would be pleased to conclude this paper by presenting research that directly evaluates the ideas offered. However, the literature on Holland's theory lacks attempts to extend his typology to predicting outcomes in interpersonal contexts. A recent study by Cox and Thoreson (1977) was the only study located that tested Holland's congruence notion in client/counselor matching. Generally, their results were equivocal for preference of similar/dissimilar counselor personality characteristics. Unfortunately, they did not include subjects' degree of self-definition (for example, consistency and differentiation) in their analysis of Holland personality types which would increase the value of their findings. Also, their definition of environments via the type of vocational activities stressed by the counselor differs somewhat from how client/counselor interaction is conceptualized in this paper. The author's application of Holland's typology to assessment of marital interaction has yielded some supportive evidence for the ideas presented. Bruch and Gilligan (1978, Note 1) found that individuals possessing higher degrees of both spouse congruence and self-definition (for example, high consistency plus high differentiation) versus those with low degrees on both factors reported significantly more positive scores on three of five measures of marital behavior employed in the study. Since counseling is often concerned with client adjustment in school, occupational, and marriage and family roles, one value in studying degree of person/environment congruence on outcomes of dyadic interaction other than counseling is to provide increasing congruence between person to person or between the person and the learning process to improve adjustment.

Hopefully, the application of Holland's typology to counselors' interaction with men discussed in this article has sensitized the reader to a number of issues and alternative considerations. There is little doubt that many men are unwilling to seek or reluctant to continue with counseling because at best they are receiving round pegs when they are square holes. While there is heterogeneity among counselors' personality styles, I feel that individually and as a profession we often construct the counseling process in our own image. S type counselors value and emphasize communication processes and skills. ISA experimental-clinical psychologists emphasize systematic cognitive-behavior modification procedures. Perhaps, more EAS and ES type counselors prefer private practice to doing systematic evaluation on the effectiveness of the techniques they employ.[1] Holland's hexagonal model should sensitize us to the need for starting with the male client's dominant personality type rather than with our own when designing and prescribing treatments for males. We need to develop alternate behavior change philosophies and methods that are especially sensitive to the socialization history and role conditioning of R, C, and some I type males. Finally, the typology suggests that current approaches to goal-setting and criteria of treatment success or failure need to consider the client's enduring personality type and the primary environment type within which he resides.

REFERENCE NOTE

1. Bruch, M. A., & Gilligan, J. F. *Extension of Holland's theory to assessment of marital interaction.* Unpublished manuscript, Bradley University, 1978.

REFERENCES

Bem, S. L. The measurement of psychological androgyny. *Journal of Consulting and Clinical Psychology*, 1974, *42*, 155–162.
Bem, S. L. On the utility of alternative procedures for assessing psychological androgyny. *Journal of Consulting and Clinical Psychology*, 1977, *45*, 196–205.
Bergin, A. L., & Garfield, S. L. (Eds.). *Handbook of psychotherapy and behavior change.* New York: Wiley, 1971.
Carkhuff, R. R. *Helping and human relations* (Vol. I & Vol II). New York: Holt, Rinehart & Winston, 1969.
Carkhuff, R. R., & Alexik, M. Effect of client depth of self-exploration upon high and low functioning counselors. *Journal of Counseling Psychology*, 1967, *14*, 350–355.
Cox, J. G., & Thoreson, R. W. Client-counselor matching: A test of the Holland model. *Journal of Counseling Psychology*, 1977, *24*, 158–161.

[1]Please excuse my implied prejudice toward particular Holland personality types, a danger pointed out by Hollifeld (1971), who I assume is Holland writing under a pen name.

Elwood, D. L. Automation methods. In F. H. Kanfer & A. P. Goldstein (Eds.), *Helping people change.* New York: Pergamon Press, 1975, 487–523.

Friel, T., Dratochevil, D., & Carkhuff, R. R. *Effect of client depth of self-exploration on therapists categorized by level of experience and type of training.* Unpublished manuscript, State University of New York at Buffalo, 1968.

Gladstein, G. A. Empathy and counseling outcome: An empirical and conceptual review. *The Counseling Psychologist,* 1977, 6(4), 70–79.

Goldstein, A. P. *Psychotherapeutic attraction.* New York: Pergamon Press, 1971.

Goldstein, A. P. *Structured learning therapy.* New York: Academic Press, 1973.

Goldstein, A. P., & Simonson, N. R. Social psychological approaches to psychotherapy research. In A. Bergan & S. Garfield (Eds.), *Handbook of psychotherapy and behavior change.* New York: Wiley, 1971, 154–195.

Gormally, J., & Hill, C. E. Guidelines for research on Carkhuff's training model. *Journal of Counseling Psychology,* 1974, 21, 539–547.

Gottfredson, G. D., & Holland, J. L. Vocational choices of men and women: A comparison of predictors from the Self-Directed Search. *Journal of Counseling Psychology,* 1975, 22, 28–34.

Hogan, R., Hall, R., & Blank, E. An extension of the similarity-attraction hypothesis to the study of vocational behavior. *Journal of Counseling Psychology,* 1972, 19, 238–240.

Holland, J. L. *Making vocational choices: A theory of careers.* Englewood Cliffs, N.J.: Prentice-Hall, 1973.

Holland, J. L., & Gottfredson, G. D. Using a typology of persons and environments to explain careers: Some extensions and clarification. *The Counseling Psychologist,* 1976, 6,(3), 20–29.

Hollifield, J. H. An extension of Holland's theory to its unnatural conclusion. *The Personnel and Guidance Journal,* 1971, 50, 209–212.

Katz, M. *System of Interactive guidance and information.* Princeton, N.J.: Educational Testing Service, 1974.

Lambert, M. J., & De Julio, S. S. Outcome research in Carkhuff's human resource development training programs: Where is the donut? *The Counseling Psychologist,* 1977, 6(4), 79–86.

Orne, M. T., & Wender, P. H. Anticipating socialization for psychotherapy: Method and rationale. *American Journal of Psychiatry,* 1968, 124, 1202–1212.

Rogers, C. R. The necessary and sufficient conditions of therapeutic personality change. *Journal of Consulting Psychology,* 1957, 22, 95–103.

Schofield, W. *Psychotherapy, the purchase of friendship.* Englewood Cliffs, N.J.: Prentice–Hall, 1964.

Schmidt, L. D., & Strong, S. R. "Expert" and "inexpert" counselors. *Journal of Counseling Psychology,* 1970, 17, 115–118.

Strong, S. R. Counseling: An interpersonal influence process. *Journal of Counseling Psychology,* 1968, 15, 215–224.

Strong, S. R., & Dixon, D. N. Expertness, attractiveness, and influence in counseling. *Journal of Counseling Psychology,* 1971, 18, 652–570.

Strong, S. R., & Matross, R. P. Change processss in counseling and psychotherapy. *Journal of Counseling Psychology,* 1973, 20, 25–37.

Strupp, H. H., & Bloxom, A. L. Preparing lower-class patients for group psychotherapy: Development and evaluation of a role-induction film. *Journal of Counseling and Clinical Psychology,* 1973, *41,* 373–384.

Truax, C. B., & Carkhuff, R. R. *Toward effective counseling and psychotherapy.* Chicago: Aldine, 1967.

Truax, C. B., & Mitchell, K. M. Research on certain therapist interpersonal skills in relation to process and outcome. In A. E. Bergin & S. L. Garfield (Eds.), *Handbook of psychotherapy and behavior change.* New York: Wiley, 1971, 154–195.

Truax, C. B., Shapiro, J. G., & Wargo, D. G. The effects of alternate sessions and vicarious therapy pretraining on group psychotherapy. *International Journal of Group Psychotherapy,* 1968, *18,* 186–198.

INTERVENTION ARTICLES 3

Academic and Behavioral Problems of Boys in Elementary School

ROBERT B. CHAPMAN
Mental Health and Mental Retardation
Authority of Harris County, Houston, Texas

ABSTRACT

The development of a boy's sex role begins shortly after birth when he is assigned certain colors due to his gender. By the time the boy is eighteen months old, adults are expecting clear sex differences in his behavior. Subtle and not so subtle pressure is put on the child to produce sex differences. The pressure is from a wide variety of sources such as type of toys purchased, clothing provided, decoration of his room, and his interactions with family members and other significant adults. Consequently the boy's preference for guns, wheeled toys, running, and aggressive play appears at or before age three. By the time the boy enters elementary school at age six, he has a strong notion of the masculine behaviors expected of him.

Modification of sex roles to accommodate the expectations of the school is one of the more difficult tasks facing elementary school aged boys. As they enter school, boys are required to assume a second role, that of a student. However, the behaviors implicit in many boys' sex roles are oppositional to the behaviors required in the student role. The conflict results in the boy not successfully assuming the student role, and may result in the boy being identified as having an academic and/or behavioral problem. Considerable research indicates that a large percentage of boys are experiencing difficulties in the schools. The present article will explore the reasons boys are involved in such frequent problems in school, and will make recommendations for persons working with elementary school aged boys.

INCIDENCE OF SCHOOL PROBLEMS

Rubin and Balow (1971) conducted a longitudinal study on 967 children whose mothers had received prenatal care and delivered in the University of Minnesota Hospital. Prior to entering school all of the subjects were screened and appeared to constitute a normal, unbiased sample of children. The childrens' teachers were asked if the children had been placed in a special class, been the recipient of special services, or identified by the teacher as having a problem with behavior or attitude. Rubin and Balow reported that 50% of the boys and 31% of the girls had been identified in one or more of the categories. Similar data were reported by Chapman, Larsen, and Parker (1978a).

Other studies on the referral rates to special services have demonstrated the magnitude of the problem. Morse, Cutler, and Fink (1964) examined the characteristics of 441 children in programs for the emotionally disturbed. They reported an age range of five to fifteen, with 9.4 years being the mean for boys. Further, they found that 83.2% of the children in these programs were male. Kvaraceus (1971) examined children who had a record with juvenile law authorities. Of all children between ages seven and nineteen, approximately 11% had a juvenile record. Eighty percent of children with a juvenile record were male.

Gilbert (1957) examined the referrals to child guidance clinics and found that boys were much more likely to experience emotional, academic, and behavioral problems. In the six to ten year old group, he found that boys constituted the vast majority of referrals for academic difficulties (74%), mental retardation (64%), aggressive and antisocial behavior (79%), passive and withdrawn behavior (70%), emotional instability and anxiety symptoms (70%), hyperactivity and motor symptoms (70%), sexual behavior problems (55%), toilet training (67%), speech defects (77%), and other miscellaneous problems (70%). Boys constituted 72% of all referrals to the clinics.

In reviewing the literature it becomes apparent that a major problem facing elementary aged boys is the control of aggression. The unusually large ratio of males referred for all types of problems leads to the speculation that misbehavior is not simply a matter of what behaviors boys exhibit, but also the manner in which adults evaluate and respond to the behaviors. That is, boys' behaviors may be evaluated more stringently by teachers and parents because of boys' characteristics. For example, boys tend to be noisier than girls. Consequently, the noise level created by a boy may call attention to his behavior and increase the probability of his behavior being identified as a problem. Further, it is interesting to note that Stone and Church (1957) state that girls' behavior is evaluated more leniently than boys. In summary, boys experience many difficulties in school. These difficulties appear to be a combination of the boy's behavior characteristics and the teacher's overreactions to certain types of behavior.

SOURCES OF SCHOOL PROBLEMS

The implicit focus of the present article is on the factors of the male sex role that result in boys experiencing problems in elementary school. As previously stated, most boys begin the first grade with a rather strong notion of the stereotyped masculine behaviors expected of them. These expectations have been molded by parents, older siblings, and other significant adults through the selection of toys, stories, idols, and interactions. For example, the toys commonly selected for boys are wheeled toys, guns, rough building blocks, footballs, and so forth, which encourage the boys to be active and assertive. Further, in play the father and siblings are rougher and play more "masculine" games with sons than daughters. The difficulty with this assertive, active, and playful style of behavior is that frequently it is considered inappropriate at school.

Elementary schoools are frequently characterized as feminized societies—that is, the system is dominated by women and reflects the norms (values, attitudes, expectations) of women. Teachers and principals are often ambivalent about the behavior of boys. They are aware that "boys will be boys," but they also feel pressure to maintain discipline and control in the classroom. The ambivalence results in the boys receiving conflicting messages about behavior and sex roles. The boys are expected to be aggressive, rough, controlling, and full of spirit while at the same time to be courteous, generous, and obedient. If the boys do not exhibit the former behaviors, adults become concerned that something is missing. If the boys do not exhibit the latter behavior they are considered to have a "problem." The "problem" may be formalized into some label of deviancy—for example, bad boy, bully, trouble maker, behavior disorder, or academic disorder.

In addition to the behavior components of boys' sex roles, there are additional differences in boys that make it difficult for them to fit into the feminized society of elementary schools. The curriculum of elementary schools is primarily concerned with the verbal spheres of learning. Boys are traditionally inferior to girls in the verbal spheres, but superior in quantitative and spatial relations. The professional interests of most elementary teachers are in the verbal sphere of languages and reading. Unfortunately the school curriculum and professional interests of teachers are directed toward girls' areas of strength and boys' areas of weakness. Not surprising, girls in general perform better school work in elementary school. The etiology of school problems has been discussed and researched for many years. Much of the work can be placed into five categories: biological factors, lack of male role models, women teachers behaving differently, teacher expectations, and the school as a feminized society.

Biological Factors

There are a number of widely held beliefs regarding biological differences in boys and girls that account for the poor performance of boys in school. Boys and girls do not differ markedly in size until age eleven. There are no differences in intellectual abilities (intelligence test scores). Around the age of six boys exhibit more physical strength and sustained energy for physical activities. The result is that boys are active, often too active, in the classroom.

A widely held belief is that boys' intelligence develops slower than girls, thus the decreased achievement in school. For example, Smith (1963) postulated that teachers are aware of developmental delays and therefore expect boys to have more difficulties in reading. More recent research has not confirmed that boys are inferior in reading skills (Broome, 1970; Cascario, 1972; Hull, 1969). The problem with boys' achievement appears to be more a matter of school curriculum and teacher interests not being consistent with that of the boys rather than a problem of delayed development.

Lack of Male Models

Benedict (1938), Kaplan (1948), Preston (1962), and others have hypothesized that boys perform poorly in school due to the absence of male teachers to act as effective role models. At present, approximately 17 % of all elementary school teachers are male (Janssen, 1977). The research on positive effects of male teachers on boys' academic performance is inconclusive. Shinedling and Pedersen (1970) found that fourth-grade males achieved more in quantitative areas with male teachers and significantly less in verbal areas with female teachers. However, contradicting evidence is presented by Davis and Slobodian (1967), Hull (1969), and Cascario (1972). The inconclusive results do not negate the concept. The research ignored more complex issues such as teacher attitude, adequacy of the male teacher as a role model, and teacher willingness to tolerate active or aggressive behavior by the boys.

The limited number of male teachers is unfortunate, since it deprives boys of male models with whom they may identify first hand. A related problem concerns the female emphasis in the curriculum, instructional materials, and books in the libraries. This problem no doubt reflects the fact that few men teach, develop educational materials, or purchase library books for elementary-aged boys.

Women Teachers Behave Differently

Women teachers respond differently to boys and girls. Further, they are often ambivalent about the boys, which results in conflicting expectations. For example, boys are expected to meet the standards of decorum laid down by females while also showing the spirit, aggressiveness, and roughness expected of males. The frustration from the conflicting messages sets the boy up to experience more problems than girls.

The major issue is whether the differential teacher behavior affects achievement. McNeil (1964) presented evidence that differential teacher behaviors had significantly lowered male students' achievements. McNeil's research methodology was criticized by Ingle and Gephart (1966) and Davis and Slobodian (1967) were unable to replicate the results.

Considerable research indicates that the boys experience different interactions with their teachers (Evertson, Brophy, & Good, 1973). The teachers initiated more interactions with the boys than girls. In turn, the boys initiated more interactions with the teachers. The boys receive many, many more criticisms and behavior warnings. The boys were in general much more active in the classroom. It may be that the high incidence of teacher-initiated interactions consisted of attempting to maintain control in the classroom. Perhaps the best interpretation of the data is that boys in general do experience different interactions with the teacher. Whether or not these differences lead to achievement or behavioral problems appears to be situation specific—that is, based on factors specific to the particular city, school, classroom, teacher, and student involved.

Teacher Expectations

The impact of teacher's expectations for a student's performance was demonstrated by Rosenthal and Jacobson (1968). They artificially increased teachers' expectations for a certain student's achievement and then observed that the student's achievement had increased. Although Rosenthal and Jacobson's work has been widely criticized and attempts to replicate it are inconclusive, the notion of teacher expectancy remains popular. For example, Palardy (1969) presented evidence that lowered teacher expectations for male achievement in reading did affect reading performance. The teachers' bias that the males would perform poorly resulted in the boys performing poorly. Antonoplos (1971) reported that teacher bias of females over males was directly transmitted to the students. The attitudes of teachers toward boys are very important, and at the extremes probably do affect achievement.

School as a Feminized Society

Educational scholars have long noted that elementary schools are designed more to meet the needs of females than males. Ayers (1909) stated, "our schools as they are now constituted are better fitted to the needs and natures of the girls than of the boys." The notion of schools as a feminized society is obviously not a new one, but more recent developments in the application of general systems theory to education and psychology do provide new understanding of the schools.

Schools are very complex social systems and exhibit the characteristics typical of all systems. One such example is homeostasis, which is a relative state of equilibrium that the system strives to maintain at all times. The defeminization of schools would pose a tremendous threat to the system's homeostatic nature. Such changes would be met with much resistance. The consequence is that certain characteristics of the system may change—for example, the boy having a male teacher—but the overall system behavior will remain essentially the same.

Another characteristic of systems concerns the roles performed by persons functioning within the system. Examples of the roles are the designated leader, the informal leader, the group conscience, the hard worker, the star, the village idiot, and the scapegoat. The roles may be performed by more than one person, and one person may move from one role to another. The roles characterized as negative—for example, trouble maker, village idiot, and scapegoat—are usually filled by boys. Once boys are entrenched in these roles it is difficult to remove them. Ebner (1967) found teachers' interventions with trouble making boys ineffective because the boys were receiving much more powerful reinforcement from their classmates for functioning in the roles. The roles performed by many boys result in their experiencing problems in the school. However, to fully appreciate the nature of the "problem" it will be necessary to understand the function of that problem within the particular system.

SOLUTIONS

This section of the paper is euphemistically entitled solutions; no single solution exists for the conflict between a boy's sex role and student role. The problems facing boys and teachers are multidimensional and very complex. The schools are in need of major revision, but the schools are not the sole perpetrators of "injustice" against young boys. The other major societal institutions—for example, family, church, business and labor, local governments, the voters, judicial systems, and the federal government—have all abdicated their responsibilities in rearing young children. The result has been increased responsibility given to the school much of which is outside of the reasonable domains of the school. The schools have become overloaded, which reduces efficiency.

The teachers and schools have no control over child characteristics that are produced in the home. Nor do they have control over chaos that occurs in the home, even though they are frequently caught in conflicts that began in the home. A classic example of this conflict is child abuse. In many states the school is required by law to report suspected child abuse. However, the parents are invariably outraged by the school's intrusion into their family matters and often attempt to intimidate or harass the school officials involved.

A boy's development of appropriate sex role is primarily determined by his home and family. With ever increasing divorce rates and "boundless" families it appears that boys will continue to have considerable difficulty in developing appropriate sex roles. The difficulties will be most noticeable in issues of authority and aggression. For example, the fantasy play of young boys normally contains much aggression, particularly of a physical nature. The degree of aggression is influenced by the boy's role models. If the boy does not have an effective adult role model to interact with on a personal basis, his role development can be inhibited.

In view of the degeneration of the family along with other societal problems, it is likely that many boys will continue to enter elementary school with poorly developed sex roles and therefore encounter academic and behavioral problems. Potential strategies for working on these problems are changes in the school, more effective methods of handling deviant classroom behavior, resolving life system problems, modifying adult sex roles, and modifying boys' sex roles.

Changes in the Schools

A word that frequently comes to mind regarding the schools is inertia. The schools have become massive bureaucracies that appear unable to move toward children's needs, or to make meaningful changes without undue delay. The need for educational reform is evident, but such reform will be slow in occurring. The observation that elementary schools are feminized societies will likely remain accurate for some time to come.

The major resource for assisting boys who are experiencing problems is the teacher. Consultation with teachers is an effective technique for bringing about situational change. Teachers are by and large competent, and delighted to have consultation about children in the classroom. Too often teachers have become the scapegoats of the ineffective educational bureaucracy. Mental health professionals have frequently held strong biases against teachers. If mental health professionals want to effectively consult with teachers, they would be wise to become sensitive to issues currently troubling teachers. Janssen (1977) states, "The psychic rewards of teaching are still unique, but layoffs and budget cuts have turned a once secure profession into a depressed industry" (p. 70). Teachers are faced with low respect for their profession, verbal and physical abuse from their students, continued shortage of operating funds, limited support from school boards, administrators, and the public at large.

A major area for consultation with teachers is the classroom as a social system. Teachers are generally unaware of the group processes operating in the classroom. They often are so busy reacting to the children's demands that they do not observe the themes in the demands or the roles being played by certain students.

Effective Methods of Handling Deviant Behavior in the Classroom

The incidence of boys' experiencing academic and behavioral problems will decrease when teachers develop a realistic expectation for boys' behavior in the classroom and have increased skills in handling deviant behavior. Teachers need specific training in conceptualizing normal and deviant behavior within the boundaries of their classrooms. All children function within the roles and boundaries of the classroom, whether their behavior is perceived to be normal or deviant. Often the positive and negative behaviors are much more similar and related than is apparent at first.

Teachers also need training in more effective methods of handling deviant behavior. Traditional strategies of handling deviant behavior may inadvertently reinforce the behavior. For example, boys designated as behavior problems are significantly more active than normal boys in the classroom (Martin, 1972). Much of this activity is disruptive to the class. Available research indicates that teachers often increase their attention as a boy increases in acting out (Chapman, Larsen, & Parker, 1979; Werry & Quay, 1969; Forness & Esveldt, 1975). Unfortunately, the strategy serves to reinforce the very behavior that was the target of control. Werry and Quay (1969) comment on this teacher behavior:

> Despite this disruptive behavior and failure to work, the deviant child nevertheless succeeded in capturing an inordinate amount of the teacher's attention which was, interestingly, mostly of a positive kind and initiated by the teacher. What these data do not show, however, is that most of this positive teacher initiated interaction occurred when the child was engaging in disruptive behavior. . . . [p. 465].

In summary, teachers need consultation and training to enable them to more effectively handle deviant behaviors in the classroom.

Resolving Life System Problems

The major life systems for elementary aged boys are the community, school, peers and family. Often the boy experiences considerable conflict between his various life systems. For example, in his community there may be a norm that school is useless or for sissys. Another common conflict is between the parents and the school, where the boy feels a pull between two strong loyalties (Coles & Piers, 1969). When the major life systems of a boy are in conflict over the boy's education, the conflict is devastating.

Change in Adult Male Sex Role

Many men are seeking new boundaries for the acceptable male sex role. They are no longer willing to accept the idea that a man's value is determined by financial success or his ability to conform to the "macho" stereotype. Men are now interested in defining their roles according to individual abilities and needs. Young boys will benefit from this redefinition, for their sex roles are based primarily on their perceptions of significant males in their lives. Sears (1953) found that warm, accepting, and rewarding fathers produce sons who are more likely to have appropriate sex-role development.

Redefine Boys' Sex Roles

The foundation for changing boys' sex roles is to change adults' sex roles. In addition, there are specific activities for skill training that may be undertaken in a school or a counseling program. These activities include new methods for relating to peers, new methods for relating to adults, redefining the limits of acceptable behavior at school, and skills expressing feelings and emotions. The ultimate goal is to reduce differences between the boy's sex role and student role which will in turn lower the frequency of boys experiencing academic and behavioral problems.

REFERENCES

Antonoplos, D. P. *Interactions of teacher-pupil sex as expressed by teacher expectations, patterns of reinforcement, and judgments about pupil: A national study.* Unpublished dissertation, Indiana University, 1971.

Ayers, L. P. *Laggards in our schools.* New York: Russell Sage Foundation, 1909.

Benedict, R. Continuities and discontinuities in cultural conditioning. *Psychiatry,* 1938, *1*, 161–167.

Broome, B. J. *An investment of the effects of teacher's expectations on the achievement in reading of first grade boys.* Unpublished dissertation, The Louisiana State University and Agricultural and Mechanical College, 1970.

Cascario, E. F. *The male teacher and reading achievement of first grade boys and girls.* Unpublished dissertation, Lehigh University, 1972.

Chapman, R. B., Larsen, S. C., & Parker, R. M. *The incidence of academic and behavioral problems in elementary schools: Replication of Rubin and Balow.* Paper presented at international Convention of the Council for Exceptional Children, May 4, 1978, Kansas City, Missouri.

Chapman, R. B., Larsen, S. C., & Parker, R. M. Interactions of first grade classroom teachers with learning disordered students. *Journal of Learning Disabilities,* 1979, *12*, 225–230.

Coles. R., & Piers, M. *Wages of neglect.* Chicago: Quadrangle Books, 1969.

Davis, O. L., & Slobodian, J. J. Teacher behavior toward boys and girls during first grade reading instruction. *American Education Research Journal,* 1967, *4*, 261–269.

Ebner, M. J. *An investigation of the role of the social environment in the generalization and persistence of the effect of a behavior modification program.* Unpublished doctoral dissertation, University of Oregon, 1967.

Evertson, C., Brophy, J., & Good, T. *Communication of teacher expectations: Second grade.* Report Series No. 92, Research and Development Center for Teacher Education, University of Texas at Austin, 1973.

Forness, S., & Esveldt, K. Classroom observations of children with learning and behavioral problems. *Journal of Learning Disabilities,* 1975, *8*(6), 382–385.

Gilbert, G. M. A survey of referral problems in Metropolitan child guidance centers. *Journal of Clinical Psychology,* 1957, *13*, 37–42.

Hull, R. E. *Sex-role identification and achievement.* Doctoral dissertation, The University of New Mexico, 1969.

Ingle, R. B., & Gephart, W. J. A critique of a research report: Programmed instruction versus usual classroom procedures in teaching boys to read. *American Educational Research Journal,* 1966, *3*, 49–53.

Janssen, P. A. Hard times in the classroom. *Money,* June 1977, 70–74.

Kaplan, L. The status and function of men teachers in urban elementary schools. *Journal of Educational Research,* 1948, *41*, 703–709.

Kvaraceus, W. C. *Prevention and control of delinquency: The school counselor's role.* Boston: Houghton Mifflin, 1971.

Martin, R. P. Student sex and behavior as determinants of the type and frequency of teacher-student contacts. *Journal of School Psychology,* 1972, *10*, 339–347.

McNeil, J. D. Programmed instruction versus visual classroom procedures in teaching boys to read. *American Educational Research Journal,* 1964, *1*, 113–119.

Morse, W. C., Cutler, R. L., & Fink, A. H. *Public school classes for the emotionally handicapped: A research analysis.* Arlington, Virginia: The Council on Exceptional Children, 1964.

Palardy, J. M. For Johnny's reading sake. *The Reading Teacher,* 1969, *22*, 721–724.

Preston, R. C. Reading achievement of German and American children. *School and Society,* 1962, *90*, 350–354.

Rosenthal, R., & Jacobson, L. *Pygmalion in the classroom: Teacher expectation and pupil intellectual development.* New York: Holt, Rinehart & Winston, 1968.

Rubin, R., & Balow, B. Learning and behavioral disorders: A longitudinal study. *Exceptional Children,* 1971, *38*(4), 293–299.

Sears, P. S. Child-rearing factors related to playing of sex-typed roles. *American Psychologist,* 1953, *8*, 431.

Shinedling, M. M., & Pedersen, D. M. Effects of sex of teacher and student on children's gain in quantitative and verbal performances. *The Journal of Psychology,* 1970, *76*, 79–84.

Smith, N. B. *Reading instruction for today's children.* Englewood Cliffs: Prentice-Hall, 1963.

Stone, L. J., & Church, J. *Childhood and adolescence.* New York: Random House, 1957.

Werry, J. S., & Quay, H. C. Observing the classroom behavior of elementary school children. *Exceptional Children,* 1969, *35*, 461–470.

Counseling-Psychotherapy and Black Men

JAMES E. SAVAGE, JR.
YVONNE KELLEY,
Howard University

As America approaches the 21st century, the ideology of America is still a profession of equality and freedom for all its members. However, any examination of the mental health of the Black man has to begin with harsh societal realities which have become common knowledge.

In the realm of work, unemployment and meaningless jobs run rampant among Black men. Quality of life, especially in terms of practical issues, serves as a touchstone for understanding men within the Black community.

The present paper explores the impact of counseling-psychotherapy or therapeutic psychology (Brammer & Shostrom, 1977) on the well-being and social effectiveness of Black men. We will proceed from a historical perspective discussing (a) the extent to which institutions and individuals diagnose and apply therapeutic psychology to the problems of Black men; (b) the utilization of existing therapeutic services by Black men; and (c) the ways cultural nuances and race are implicated in the application of therapeutic psychology. Finally, ways in which training in therapeutic psychology can be improved to meet the needs of the Black man are discussed.

HISTORICAL PERSPECTIVE

The incessant struggle by the Black man to gain full membership status in American society has been extensively documented (Cuban 1964; DuBois, 1903/1961; Ebony, 1971; Frazier, 1970; Hamilton, 1976; Lyons, 1971; Meier & Rudwick, 1974; Quarles, 1964). The extent to which the Black man's consistent push toward equality and freedom has been thwarted by a continuous pattern of discriminatory and racist behavior is also documented (J.H. Franklin, 1969; Jones, 1972; Gossett, 1965; Segal, 1967; Stephenson, 1910/1969; Waskow, 1967).

Historically, a systematic set of intergroup relationships exist between the Black community and the larger White society that influence the (a) beliefs and values of both groups; (b) amount and quality of reality testing engaged in by each about the other; and (c) many negative feelings each holds for the other. As a result, it has been the Black community which has historically encountered—because of its subordinate status—the external pressures from the wider society. These pressures have been disruptive and have led to high levels of disorganizing stress and strain within the Black community, family, and individual. Recent data reported by the U.S. Department of Health, Education and Welfare (Note 1) show that (a) Blacks have less education, more unemployment, and less income than Whites; (b) Blacks are more likely than Whites to come from a large female-headed family that is poor; (c) the percentage of Blacks living in crowded conditions and poor housing is 2–3 times higher than the percentage of Whites living in such conditions; and (d) Blacks experience more sickness, disability, and violent death than Whites. Moreover, this same document reported that the number of Blacks housed in penal facilities was over nine times greater than the number of Whites; in mental hospitals, Black patients were reported to outnumber Whites by 52%.

Another report by Rose (1971) emphasized the vulnerability of Blacks to various dangers in their present eco-system. *Ecosystem,* for the purpose of this paper, is defined as the personal and impersonal environment of the Black man, which is comprised of family (present and absent), community (Black people, things, and institutional symbols such as the Black church), and the wider society (that is, White people, things, and institutions). The history of the Black man in America lends strong support to the notion that he has little reason for experiencing ecosystem trust-control, which is the belief that the ecological forces in his environment are favorable and controllable, especially as they relate to him maintaining a high quality of life and ecological balance. Too many Black men experience ecosystem distrust-noncontrol (that is, the belief that forces within the ecological system are detrimental to them in maintaining a high quality of life, ecological balance, and control).

Some historical antecedents that have led to much ecosystem distrust-noncontrol among Black males are still prevalent and have grave implication for Black males' sense of worth and prerogatives. These forces also impact upon those institutions and individuals who utilize therapeutic psychology on the behalf of the Black male.

IMPLICATIONS FOR DIAGNOSIS AND COUNSELING-PSYCHOTHERAPY

Those who make diagnoses and provide counseling-psychotherapy must take into account both the Black man's psychological and political needs. In terms of a hierarchy of needs, his self-actualization is inversely related to his continued subjugation and oppression. The possession of basic human rights is imperative if the Black man is to experience total mental health. Therefore, most aspects of therapeutic psychology applied to the problems of the Black man should be proactive rather than reactive (Allport, 1962). Otherwise, this psychology becomes what Kennedy and Kerber (1973, p.39) define as resocialization, which is:

> that process wherein an individual defined as inadequate according to the norms of a dominant institution(s), is subjected to a dynamic program of behavior intervention aimed at installing and/or rejuvenating those values, attitudes, and abilities which would allow him to function according to the norms of said dominant institution(s).

Historically, therapeutic psychology for the Black man has been for the primary purpose of resocialization. This is carried out in programs of compensatory education, mental health, and criminal rehabilitation for maintainance of the status quo (Lerner, 1972; Roberts, Savage, & Adair, Note 2; Thomas & Sillen, 1972).

Within the context of resocialization, Blacks are diagnosed differently than Whites. At a young age they are more likely to be labelled EMR and hyperactive (Williams, 1977). At an older age, even when controlling for social class, they are more often diagnosed schizophrenic than White men of this age group (Morton, Rosen, & Willis, Note 3; Simpson, Note 1; Cannon & Locke, Note 4). Because the Black man so often receives therapeutic psychology in the context of resocialization, he is resculptured, usually into a politically powerless individual, with less ecosystem trust-control. It is little wonder that many Black males fail to utilize existing therapeutic services.

UTILIZATION OF MENTAL HEALTH SERVICES

The various external pressures that impact upon the Black man and the many stresses and strains he experiences, both interpersonally and intrapersonally, place him at the highest risk of experiencing psychological distress. Yet, many Black men do not seek counseling-psychotherapy until they get feedback from their ecosystem that they are intolerably out of kilter. Their behavior is usually reported to the police. The legal system then becomes the leading source of referral of Black men to state and county mental hospitals (Cannon & Locke, Note 4).

Various reasons have been posited as to why the Black male delays his first visit or admission to outpatient facilities and other counseling services (cf., Cannon & Locke, Note 4; See & Miller, 1973). Personal observation and reflection of the literature have stimulated the following postulate:

1. There exists an inverse relationship between the Black man who is at highest risk of experiencing psychological distress and the quantity and/or quality of therapeutic services available to him.

? There exists a significant inverse relationship between the Black man who is the highest utilizer of public and/or government-funded mental health facilities and the number of therapeutic psychologists who are of the same race and sex as himself.

3. To the extent that more reliable therapeutic services are provided and the number of Black psychologists are significantly increased within the ecosystem of the Black man, he will experience increased ecosystem trust-control and the latency of this first visit or admission to mental health facilities will decrease.

4. As (3) becomes a reality, there will be less reliance by the Black man upon untrained communal counselors-psychotherapists, hard drugs, and alcohol to maintain ecosystem balance.

For example, the World Community of Islam in the West, formerly the Nation of Islam, has implemented a variety of programs that relate to the postulates listed above. Their counseling methods have had many positive results in "prohabilitating" men who were institutionalized for various crimes and vices. Their methods have also prevented many Black men from becoming emotionally unstable.

The postulates are stated on a macro-level. Equally important are the transactions that occur on a micro-level within therapeutic psychology— that is, the therapeutic relationship.

RACE AND THE THERAPEUTIC RELATIONSHIP

There have been many discussions by therapeutic psychologists and others as to the negative and/or positive effects of race and culture in the therapeutic relationship. Reviews of this body of literature have been presented by See and Miller (1973) and Sattler (1970). Their papers seem to suggest that most findings regarding the effects of the race of therapists are equivocal. However, Sattler points out that the more contemporary studies show a need for matching the therapeutic psychologist and his/her client by race. He also indicates that more research must be done in this area.

Recent writings also show that there are distinct linguistic differences that exist between Black men and White men born out of different cultural experiences (Andrews & Owens, 1973; Hall & Freedle, 1975; Kochman, 1972; Landis, McGraw, Day, Savage, & Saral, 1976; Williams, 1977). These differences can be barriers to establishing the rapport needed for an effective therapeutic relationship.

For example, pilot data from research that we are in the process of completing show that, when White and Black college students were asked to free associate for one minute to the words *me* and *education,* significant variation occurred between Blacks and Whites. Additional words that were used also produced significant differences.

Other writers have reported race bias that exists in psychological tests (Dixon, 1977; Williams, 1977), test administration (A. J. Franklin,

1977; Savage, in press), and the diagnostic system (Savage & Adair, 1977). Proper diagnosis of the Black man with valid and reliable assessment tools should be primary and imperative as a goal of therapeutic psychology.

Therapeutic psychology, if it is to serve the Black man effectively, must embrace his subjective culture. "Subjective culture is a cultural group's characteristic way of viewing the man-made part of the environment" (Triandis, 1976, p. 11). The Black man's subjective culture has been greatly influenced by his experience in America, which has many facets to it that must be understood in terms of their historical antecedent in Africa (Ford, 1939; Herskovits, 1958), on this continent (Young, 1972), and in the Black community (Savage & Tapley, 1976). There is some overlap between the subjective culture of Whites and the subjective culture of Blacks; it is upon this shared set of experiences that White therapeutic psychologists and the Black man can make choices that have not been possible before. Otherwise, the cultural differences that are extant for both will widen the gulf between mainly White therapeutic psychologists, who to a great extent are rooted in traditionality, and the contemporary Black man.

In recent years, many voices have called for more relevant counseling of Blacks who are disadvantaged (Adkins, 1970; Bancroft, 1967; Maynard & Hansen, 1970; McGrew, 1971; Smith, Barnes, & Scales, 1974) and Black young adults (Vontress, 1967, Note 5, Note 6). Some writers have even suggested that Whites cannot adequately counsel the Black man (Williams & Kirkland, 1971), while others disagree with reservations that Whites cannot be effective counsellors with the Black man (Rousseve, 1970; Vontress, 1971). Since history, culture, and race have been shown to some extent to influence the therapeutic relationship (Sattler, 1970), recommendations are in order for those who practice therapeutic psychology with the Black man. These are reported below.

RECOMMENDATIONS

For effective therapeutic psychology with the Black man, the psychologist must first prepare himself structurally, that is, he/she must adopt or possess a system of values and beliefs that will facilitate the Black male's expression of ecosystem trust-control. Naturally, the psychologist must be aware of the basic tools of therapeutic psychology. Additional knowledge related to the history and experience of the Black male should be acquired through training (Harper, 1973). Moreover, the psychologist must be genuine in his behavior in order to (a) avoid stereotyped feelings, (b) be intuitive, and (c) maximize creativity. By achieving mental soundness, the psychologist minimizes or eliminates any personal communication that can produce more ecosystem distrust-noncontrol for the Black man.

Second, the therapeutic psychologist must be able to give, accept, ask for, and set limits genuinely and realistically (that is, not permitting the Black man to use his blackness as a crutch) during his therapeutic involvement with the Black man. The psychologist, when appropriate, must be able to compliment and/or offer constructive criticism. Information and other objective data should be communicated to the Black man. Communiques of empathy and/or humor should also be expressed.

Third, the psychologist must, during the time allowed, authentically engage the Black man in therapeutic activities that move him toward ecosystem trust-control. Authentic involvement means utilizing time devoid of estrangement, routine, idle chatter, unplanned tasks, and double talk. The therapist must facilitate the Black man's genuine involvement in mutually agreeable tasks directed at achieving the desired therapeutic goals and objectives within a reasonable period of time.

Fourth, the psychologist's goal should be to facilitate the Black male's development and refinement of social skills necessary to transact with elements in his ecosystem. Communicative ability is necessary for ecological balance, inasmuch as good interpersonal relationships are of paramount importance for the Black male, both psychologically and politically.

Fifth, the therapeutic psychologist should be skilled in working effectively with the Black male in improving his basic feeling of self-esteem and the esteem he holds toward elements within his ecosystem by supplying information regarding the racial myths that exist in the wider society and influence the self-esteem of the Black man. Ecosystem trust-control is directly related to the person's feeling of worth and the value he accords others. Psychologists, performing counseling-psychotherapy should understand Cross' developmental stages of Black Nigrescence (Williams, 1977), which are closely tied to the esteem of the Black male and the esteem he holds for others within his ecosystem. These stages that the Black man may undergo are:

Stage 1: Pre-Encounter. In this stage, a person thinks, acts, and behaves in a manner that degrades Blackness.

Stage 2: Encounter. The Black person becomes extremely motivated to search for Black identity.

Stage 3: Immersion-Emersion. The person develops a sense of Black pride, sports an Afro-hairstyle, wears African-inspired clothing, takes an African name, and becomes an "Afro-American," "Black," or "Black American." Confrontation is the primary form of communication.

Stage 4: Internalization. The Black person achieves a feeling of inner security, is more satisfied with him- or herself, and is more receptive to meaningful changes in his or her world-view.

Sixth, the therapeutic psychologist should be willing to serve as a political advocate for his/her Black male client especially as it relates to combatting psychosocial forces that are impacting upon the Black male and causing ecosystem imbalance. These external forces strongly influence the future goals and plans that the Black male has and wants to see unfold. When personal life plans are stymied, it creates ecosystem distrust-noncontrol. Gunnings (Note 7) says that a psychologist must counsel and deliver psychotherapy systematically; that is, the therapist must be willing to negotiate with various social systems that may be impeding the progress of his/her client.

Last, the therapeutic psychologist must shift away from value-free counseling-psychotherapy toward counseling-psychotherapy that questions social conditions. Specifically, the therapist must accept and deal with the problems of the Black man. Problem solving should be integrative—building on the strength of the Black man. This means the therapist must be able to accept interdependence, participate in a team approach, and permit mutual goal setting. This approach to counseling-psychotherapy allows the Black man to develop and/or increase substantially ecosystem trust-control.

REFERENCE NOTES

1. Simpson, Clay E., Jr. *Health of the disadvantaged chartbook* (Report No. [HRA] 77–628). Hyattsville, Md.: U. S. Department of Health, Education, and Welfare, Health Resources Administration, September, 1977.
2. Roberts, A., Savage, J. E., Jr., & Adair, A. V. *Black mental health.* Washington: Howard University, The Institute for Urban Affairs and Research, October, 1976.
3. Morton, K., Rosen, B. M., & Willis, E. M. *Definitions and distributions of mental disorders in a racist society.* Rockville, Md.: U.S. Department of Health, Education, and Welfare Public Health Service, n.d.
4. Cannon, M. S., & Locke, B. Z. *Being Black is detrimental to one's mental health: Myth or reality?* Paper presented at the meeting of the W. E. B. DuBois Conference on the Health of Black Populations, Atlanta, December, 1976.
5. Vontress, C. E., *Counseling the Black and Puerto Rican college student.* New York: Queens College Press, 1972.
6. Vontress, C. E., *First national conference on counseling minorities and disadvantaged.* East Lansing, Mich.: Michigan State Press, 1973.
7. Gunnings, T. S. *A systematic approach to counseling.* Unpublished manuscript, Michigan State University, 1976.

REFERENCES

Adkins, W. R. Life skills: Structured counseling for the disadvantaged. *Personnel and Guidance Journal,* 1970, *49,* 108–116.
Allport, G. W. Psychological models for guidance. *Harvard Educational Review,* 1962, *32,* 373–381.
Andrews, M., & Owens, P. T. *Black language.* Berkeley: Seymour-Smith, 1973.
Bancroft, J. F. Counseling the disadvantaged child. *School Counselor,* 1967, *14,* 149–156.

Brammer, I. M., & Shootrom, E. L. *Therapeutic psychology: Fundamentals of counseling and psychotherapy*. Englewood Cliffs, N.J.: Prentice-Hall, 1977.

Cuban, L. *The Negro in America*. Glenview, IL: Scott & Foresman, 1964.

Dixon, N. R. (Ed.). Testing Black students. *The Negro Educational Review*, 1977, *28*, 137–239.

DuBois, W. E. B. *The souls of Black folk*. New York: Fawcett, 1961. (Originally published, 1903.)

The editors of Ebony. *Ebony pictorial history of Black America* (3 vols.). Chicago: Johnson, 1971.

Ford, T. P. *God wills the Negro*. Chicago: The Geographical Institute Press, 1939.

Franklin, A. J. What clinicians should know about testing Black students. *The Negro Educational Review*, 1977, *28*, 202–218.

Franklin, J. H. (Ed.). *Color and race*. Boston: Beacon Press, 1969.

Frazier, T. R. *Afro-American history: Primary sources*. New York: Harcourt, Brace & World, 1970.

Gossett, T. F. *Race: The history of an idea in America*. New York: Schochen Books, 1965.

Hall, W. S., & Freedle, R.O. *Culture and language: The Black American experience*. New York: Halstead Press, 1975.

Hamilton, C. V. *The struggle for political equality*. Washington, D.C.: National Urban League, 1976.

Harper, F. D. What counselors must know about the social sciences of Black Americans. *Journal of Negro Education*, 1973, *42*, 109–116.

Herskovits, M. J. *The myth of the Negro past*. Boston: Beacon Press, 1958.

Jones, J. M. *Prejudice and racism*. Reading, Mass.: Addison-Wesley, 1972.

Kennedy, D. B., & Kerber, A. *Resocialization: An American experiment*. New York: Behavioral Publications, 1973.

Kochman, T. *Rappin' and stylin' out: Communication in urban Black America*. Urbana: University of Illinois Press, 1972.

Landis, D., McGrew, P., Day, H., Savage, J., & Saral, T. Word meanings in Black and White. In H. C. Triandis (Ed.), *Variations in Black and White perceptions of the social environment*. Urbana: University of Illinois Press, 1976.

Lerner, B. *Therapy in the ghetto: Political impotence and personal disintegration*. Baltimore: The Johns Hopkins University Press, 1972.

Lyons, T. T. *Black leadership in American history*. Reading, Mass.: Addison-Wesley, 1971.

Maynard, P. E., & Hansen, J. C. Vocational maturity among inner-city youths. *Counseling Psychology*, 1970, *17*, 400–404.

McGrew, J. M. Counseling the disadvantaged child: A practice in search of a rationale. *School Counselor*, 1971, *18*, 165–176.

Meier, A., & Rudwick, E. *The making of Black America* (2 vols.). New York: Atheneum, 1974.

Quarles, B. *The Negro in the making of America*. New York: Collier, 1964.

Rose, H. M. *The Black ghetto: A spatial behavioral perspective*. New York: McGraw-Hill, 1971.

Rousseve, R. Reason and reality in counseling the student-client who is Black. *The School Counselor*, 1970, *17*, 337–344.

Sattler, J. Racial "experimenter effects" in experimentation, testing, interviewing, and psychotherapy. *Psychological Bulletin*, 1970, *73*, 137–160.

Savage, J. E., Jr. Tester's influence on children's intellectual performance: A multivariate approach. *Journal of Negro Education*, in Press.

Savage, J. E., Jr., & Adair, A. V. Testing minorities: Developing more culturally relevant assessment systems. *The Negro Educational Review*, 1977, *28*, 219–228.

Savage, J. E., Jr., & Tapley, R. The dozens. *Transactional Analysis Journal*, 1976, *6*, 18–20.

See, J. J., & Miller, K. S. Mental health. In K. S. Miller & R. M. Dreger (Eds.), *Comparative studies of Blacks and Whites in the United States*. New York: Seminar Press, 1973.

Segal, R. *The race war*. New York: Bantam, 1967.

Smith, G. S., Barnes, E., & Scales, A. Counseling the Black child. *Elementary School Guidance and Counseling*, 1974, *8*, 245–253.

Stephenson, G. T. *Race distinctions in American law*. New York: Negro Universities Press, 1969. (Originally published, 1910.)

Thomas, A., & Sillen, S. *Racism and psychiatry*. New York: Brunner/Mazel, 1972.

Triandis, H. C. (Ed.). *Variations in Black and White perceptions of the social environment*. Urbana: University of Illinois Press, 1976.

Vontress, C. E. Counseling Negro adolescents. *School Counselor*, 1967, *15*, 86–91.

Vontress, C. E. Racial differences: Impediments to progress. *Journal of Counseling Psychology*, 1971, *18*, 7–13.

Waskow, A. I. *From race riot to sit-in: 1919 and the 1960s*. Garden City, New York: Anchor, 1967.

Williams. R. L. *Psychological tests and minorities*. (DHEW Publication No. [ADM] 77–482, U.S. Government Printing Office Stock No. 017–024–00656–4.) Washington, D.C.: U.S. Government Printing Office, 1977.

Williams, R. L., & Kirkland, J. A. The White counselor and the Black client. *The Counseling Psychologist*, 1971, *2*(4), 114–117.

Young, C. *Black experience: Analysis and synthesis*. San Rafael, Calif.: Leswing Press, 1972.

Sex Offenders: Clinical Characteristics and Treatment Methods

MICHAEL D. STOCKTON
DENISE EDWARDS
BRAINARD HINES
North Florida Evaluation and Treatment Center
Gainesville, Florida

One of the most rapidly increasing needs in counseling with men is the development of practical and effective treatment methods for individuals who display deviant sexual behavior. Included in this category are the acts of rape, pedophilia (child molestation), incest, exhibitionism, voyeurism, and fetishism. Of these offenses, rape has received the most attention from the scientific and clinical community. This may be primarily attributable to the fact that rape is the most rapidly increasing crime of violence in America and to an increased public awareness of rape as a consequence of the women's movement (Brownmiller, 1975). It should be noted that persons committing nonassaultive sex offenses, such as child molestation and exhibitionism, are more frequently referred for treatment than are rapists (Kusuda, Note 1; MacDonald & Williams, Note 2). Therefore, the problems common to a variety of sex offenders need to be considered in treatment planning.

Traditionally, counseling of sex offenders has occurred within the context of inpatient settings, usually associated with a state prison or mental hospital (Brecher, 1977). The predominance of inpatient treatment facilities for sex offenders is largely due to the enactment of sexual psychopath laws in a number of states during the late 1940s and early 1950s. Such laws, many of which are in effect today, define almost all convicted sex offenders as deranged, with rehabilitation being a secondary or nonexistent consideration (Gebhard, Gagnon, Pomeroy, & Christenson, 1965). More recent legislation in some states—for example, Florida and California—has provided for the establishment of specialized inpatient facilities for court-referred sex offenders (Stockton, Legum, &

McAnaney, 1978) as well as outpatient programs for nonviolent sex offenders as the least restrictive treatment alternative (Giarretto, 1976).

The current emphasis on the rehabilitation of sex offenders has led to the development of several innovative and promising treatment methods to meet the diverse needs of this population. To facilitate effective treatment planning, the present article will survey the clinical characteristics of sex offenders, review current therapeutic methods, and propose a treatment strategy.

CLINICAL CHARACTERISTICS

To develop an adequate strategy for treating sex offenders, it is necessary to have some knowledge of their specific clinical characteristics. Most studies assessing sex offenders have examined rather general demographic and personality attributes (Amir, 1971; Gebhard et al., 1965; Kusuda, Note 1; MacDonald & Williams, Note 2). From these data the profile of the "typical" sex offender which emerges may be described as follows:

> The sex offender is likely to be a caucasian, semi-skilled worker between the ages of 20 and 35. Generally, he has exhibited no previous deviant sexual behavior other than the present offense, although he may have frequently committed other crimes of a trivial nature. He has usually had an active sex life at some time and he is often married with children. Socially and psychologically, he is a "loner" with limited social skills and meager interpersonal relationships. He harbors deep rooted feelings of inadequacy and inferiority, an obvious dynamic in his expressed need to dominate, overpower, or humiliate his victim. His preference is for a victim younger than himself, often a pre-pubescent female, with whom he feels more secure and less threatened than with an adult female. He is typically of above average intelligence but he is an underachiever in terms of education and vocational accomplishment. He probably has a history of alcohol dependency and was drinking at the time of his offense. As is true of the alcohol prone individual, his home life is marred with conflict and disruption of the family unit. His divorce rate is approximately three to four times that of the general population.

A profile of the "typical" sex offender may have treatment implications for a heterogeneous group of sex offenders. However, a more specific clinical description of the sex offender is necessary for individualized treatment planning. In this regard, it will be useful to compare two contrasting types of sex offenders, rapists and pedophiles, providing a case study of each.

Frequently, rapists have been found to display aggressive, antisocial features, often having histories of other criminal or violent behavior (Amir, 1971; Henn, Herjanic, & Vanderpearl, 1976; MacDonald & Williams,

Note 2). In contrast, pedophiles tend to be more passive, childlike, and inadequate individuals (Henn et al., 1976; Pacht & Cowden, 1974; Glueck, Note 3). As a group rapists are youthful, usually under the age of 30, while pedophiles span a wide age range, including many elderly men (DeFrancis, 1969; Henn et al., 1976; Mohr, Turner, & Jerry, 1964). Rapists typically victimize adult females, with an underlying motive to control, dominate, or humiliate their victims, (Groth, Burgess, & Holstrom, 1977). Pedophiles select children as their victims, generally due to a fear of adult relationships, particularly with females (Bell & Hall, 1971).

The case of Mr. A., 29 years of age, illustrates many of the features of an aggressive rapist:

> Mr. A. is a highly perfectionistic, rigid, paranoid individual who married a girl 10 years his junior following a stormy and unsuccessful first marriage. After finding his wife unfaithful, Mr. A. began drinking heavily and driving the streets looking for her. Upon seeing a lone woman who resembled his wife, Mr. A. threatened her with a pistol, forcing her into his car where he beat and raped her. Several similar rape episodes continued over a period of approximately two years before Mr. A. was identified by one of his victims and arrested. Each of Mr. A's rapes was precipitated by suspicions of his wife and each rape allowed him to establish control, displace hostility, and reinforce his masculinity. Also each rape was accompanied by alcohol consumption and homocidal fantasies.

Mr. B., a 43-year-old pedophile, displays many of the inadequate features common to this type of offender:

> A shy, withdrawn individual, Mr. B. came from a home controlled by a domineering and seductive mother. He was not allowed to date until he was in his twenties, and was punished for all attempts at heterosexual contact. He was not permitted to assert himself at any time during his childhood or adolescence or to question the decisions made by his parents for him. Consequently, Mr. B. became a socially inadequate, timid individual who had a negative opinion of his abilities as a male, and whose only successful relationships were with children. Mr. B. began having sexual relations with the children of his friends at age 29 and continued these offenses over a 14 year period. He admits to planning these activities and to actually seducing the children.

Despite the apparent clinical differences between the rapist and the pedophile, these men present a number of characteristics common to many sex offenders. Both have poor self-concepts, including serious doubts about their masculinity; both had poor heterosexual relationships prior to their offense; and both lack adequate social skills and the ability to express their feelings assertively.

Thus, it can be seen that these individuals have a variety of treatment needs which must be addressed for effective rehabilitation. Besides the necessity for uncovering the motivation for their deviant sexual acts, they need to develop the skills necessary to acquire and maintain an appropriate heterosexual relationship in society. They also need to learn to express themselves in an assertive manner, rather than behaving hostilely as is true of the rapist or passively as exemplified by the pedophile.

Treatment methods which address the needs of sex offenders are employed in a variety of inpatient and oupatient settings. The following section will discuss these methods as they relate to the counseling of sex offenders.

TREATMENT METHODS

Most therapists who treat sex offenders rely on a variety of therapeutic approaches to modify deviant sexual behavior. Some of the current treatment methods are group psychotherapy, social/sexual skills training, behavior therapy, "self-help" or peer counseling, sex education, empathy training, and family therapy.

Group psychotherapy is typically the primary therapeutic modality in the treatment of sex offenders (Brecher, 1977). The group model, which is an efficient and practical treatment method, is based on the assumption that sexual deviancy has its roots in interpersonal dynamics. A social setting is then presumed necessary to alter maladaptive patterns of relating to other people. The primary function of a sex offender therapy group is to have offenders confront each other with regard to specific problems that led to their offense, to accept responsibility for their deviant sexual behavior, to develop insight into the nature and causes of their interpersonal difficulties, and to acquire new and socially acceptable sexual behavior patterns.

Another common mode of treatment used with sex offenders is social/sexual skills training, the goal of which is to increase interpersonal effectiveness, particularly with females (Abel, Blanchard, & Becker, 1976; McDonald, 1974; Boozer, Note 4). The rationale for such training is that, while the offender may be attracted to and aroused by sexual partners, he will not be able to develop an appropriate sexual relationship unless he learns preliminary conversation, flirting, and other dating skills. Social/sexual skills training requires utilization of a female therapist for the purpose of role playing, modeling, and practicing social behaviors with the offender.

Many clinicians place emphasis on social learning theory and behavior therapy (Abel, Blanchard, & Becker, 1977). The behavioral approaches are designed to alter learning patterns which develop and maintain deviant sexual behavior, to extinguish deviant sexual arousal, and/or to increase appropriate sexual arousal. Covert sensitization, fading, and/orgasmic conditioning are methods used to modify maladaptive sexual fantasies and behaviors (Abel, Blanchard, Barlow, & Flanagan, 1975; Abel & Blanchard, 1974; Marshall, 1973). The premise underlying these approaches is that sex offenders, particularly rapists, are overaroused to deviant sexual stimuli and underaroused to appropriate sexual stimuli (Abel, Barlow, Blanchard, & Guild, 1977).

A therapeutic approach which has gained increasing attention recently is the self-help treatment model developed at South Florida State Hospital (Boozer, Note 4) and at Western State Hospital in Washington (McDonald, 1974). In a self-help program, offenders assume primary responsibility for their own treatment. As offenders demonstrate progress, they adopt leadership roles in group psychotherapy, peer counseling, and ward government activities. The staff generally function as consultants to the group either through direct presence as observers in therapy sessions or through progress reports and supervisory sessions with group leaders. Self-help treatment is economical in terms of treatment resources and reduced client/therapist dependency.

Other therapists (Brancale, Virocola, & Prendergast, 1972; Burkhardt, Note 5; Seely, Note 6) emphasize sex education as a major component of treatment. The premise of sex education is that many sex offenders lack fundamental knowledge of even the simplest facts concerning human sexuality and are ingrained with deeply puritanical sexual attitudes and feelings. Through sex education the offender is afforded an opportunity to exchange mythical and distorted views about sexuality for factual knowledge concerning responsible sexual attitudes and behavior.

Empathy training is a technique designed to increase the sex offenders' awareness of and regard for the feelings of victims, actual and potential (Stockton et al., 1978). During empathy training, offenders are taught basic communication and listening skills. Several procedures include active listening exercises, role-playing, and interactions with victims of sex offenses. Since a lack of empathy appears to contribute to sex offenses, most sex offenders could potentially benefit from such training.

Another approach, which has shown promise in the treatment of father/daughter incest, is family systems therapy (Giarretto, 1976). This therapeutic approach, based on the theory and methods of humanistic psychology, includes individual counseling (for the child, mother, and father), mother/daughter counseling, marital counseling, father/daughter counseling, family counseling, and group counseling. Therapy for the family members proceeds from self-assessment and confrontation to self-identification to self-management. Principal sources of the techniques utilized are psychosynthesis, Gestalt therapy, conjoint therapy, psychodrama, transactional analysis, and personal journal keeping.

Other treatment methods are sometimes used with sex offenders. These include psychoanalytic psychotherapy (Salzman, 1972), surgical castration (Stürup, 1968), androgen-depleting hormones (Money, 1970), marathon groups (Brancale et al., 1972), sensitivity training (Brancale et al., 1972), and pastoral counseling (Oates, 1972).

The treatment methods which have been described have shown promise in modifying deviant sexual behavior. However, few attempts have been made to develop reliable and valid measures of therapeutic effectiveness with sex offenders. The studies assessing treatment outcome for sex offenders have usually relied on recidivism rates, often with differential criteria—for example, rearrest, rearrest for sexual crimes, rehospitalization, and so forth. Variability also exists in the data collection procedures; some clinicians have utilized a limited follow-up period while others carry out an extensive follow-up for five years or longer. Despite these considerations, the results obtained to date suggest that, with relevant treatment, most sex offenders have a low recidivism rate, typically ranging from 0 to 9% (Abel et al., 1976).

One strategy currently being developed to assess treatment outcome with rapists relies on multiple procedures (Abel, 1976). The evaluation process involves subdividing sexually deviant behavior into four major components: "(1) the extent of deviant arousal, (2) the amount of heterosexual arousal, (3) the adequacy of heterosocial skills, and (4) the appropriateness of gender role behavior." Three methods are recommended to assess each of the components: self-report of deviant fantasies and behaviors, physiological arousal to sexual stimuli, and behavioral observation in social situations. Although it may not be feasible to employ extensive assessment procedures in all therapeutic situations with sex offenders, evaluation of the therapy process needs to be considered as an important component of treatment. Without valid measures of therapeutic outcome, the effectiveness of the treatment method will remain unknown (Pacht, 1976).

CONCLUSION

Effective treatment planning for the sex offender requires an assessment of his clinical characteristics. A variety of interpersonal difficulties are common to many sex offenders. These include feelings of sexual inadequacy, an inability to express feelings in an open and direct manner (as opposed to aggressiveness or under-assertiveness), poor heterosexual relationships, alcohol dependency, and family conflict. In addition, differences exist among certain types of sex offenders such as rapists and pedophiles. Rapists are frequently aggressive individuals who attempt to overpower, dominate or humiliate their victims. Pedophiles tend to be passive, inadequate, immature males who select youthful victims with whom they feel more secure and less threatened than with adults.

An appropriate strategy for treating most sex offenders is an eclectic approach utilizing a variety of therapeutic techniques. An important component of treatment is group psychotherapy with the primary responsibility being placed on the offender to change his deviant sexual behavior. Assertive and social/sexual skills training utilizing a female therapist is necessary to remediate the offender's deficit in social/sexual skills. Sex education provides an appropriate modality to address the sex offender's lack of knowledge and misconceptions concerning human sexuality. For the sex offender who is overaroused to deviant sexual stimuli or underaroused to appropriate sexual stimuli, behavior therapy techniques are indicated. Empathy training is appropriate for most sex offenders because a limited awareness of and disregard for the victim's feelings seems to contribute to sex offenses. When feasible, marriage and family therapy should be an integral part of treatment because most sex offenders, particularly those involved in incestuous relationships with their children, have a disruptive family life. Often the difficulties inherent in the sex offender's family unit are related to long-term alcohol abuse. In these instances, substance abuse counseling should be provided during the course of treatment.

An often overlooked aspect of therapy with sex offenders is the systematic collection of pertinent information concerning treatment outcome. Without adequate data collection, the effectiveness of the treatment strategy employed will remain unknown. While valid measures of therapeutic effectiveness with sex offenders are still in the initial stages of development, a multimethod assessment process, including behavioral, physiological, and self-report measures, is indicated.

By assessing and treating a wide range of problems relevant to the sex offender, a viable strategy can be developed to modify deviant sexual behavior and provide the sex offender with the necessary skills for effective community living.

REFERENCE NOTES

1. Kusuda, P. *Wisconsin's first eleven years of experience with its sex crimes law.* State Department of Public Welfare, Madison, Wisconsin, April, 1965.
2. MacDonald, G., & Williams, R. *Characteristics and management of committed sexual offenders in the State of Washington.* State of Washington, Department of Social and Health Services, January 1971.
3. Glueck, B. Final Report, *Research project for the study and treatment of persons convicted of crimes involving sexual aberrations.* New York State: Department of Mental Hygiene, 1956.
4. Boozer, G. *Offender treatment: Programming (workshop).* Presented at Sixth Alabama Symposium of Justice and the Behavioral Sciences, University of Alabama, Tuscaloosa, Alabama, January, 1975.
5. Burkhardt, P. Personal communication, 1977.
6. Seely, R. Personal communication, 1977.

REFERENCES

Abel, G. G., Assessment of sexual deviation in the male. In M. Hersen & A. J. Bellack (Eds.), *Behavioral assessment: A practical handbook.* New York: Pergamon Press, 1976.

Abel, G. G., Barlow, D. H., Blanchard, E. B., & Guild, D. The components of rapists' sexual arousal. *Archives of General Psychiatry,* 1977, *34*(8), 895–903.

Abel, G. G., & Blanchard, E. B. The role of fantasy in the treatment of sexual deviation. *Archives of General Psychiatry,* 1974, *30,* 467–475.

Abel, G. G., Blanchard, E. B., Barlow, D., & Flanagan, B. *A controlled behavioral treatment of a sadistic rapist.* Paper presented at the convention of the Association for the Advancement of Behavior Therapy, San Francisco, December, 1975.

Abel, G. G., Blanchard, E. B., & Becker, J. Psychological treatment of rapists. In M. Walker & S. Brodsky (Eds.), *Sexual assault.* Lexington, Mass.: D. C. Heath, 1976.

Abel, G. G., Blanchard, E. B., & Becker, J. An integrated treatment program for rapists. In R. Rada (Ed.), *Clinical aspects of the rapist.* New York: Grune & Stratton, 1977.

Amir, M. *Patterns of forcible rape.* Chicago: University of Chicago Press, 1971.

Bell, A., & Hall, C. *The personality of a child molester: An analysis of dreams.* Chicago: Aldine & Atherton, 1971.

Brancale, R., Virocola, A., & Prendergast, W. The New Jersey program for sex offenders. In H. Resnik & M. Wolfgang (Eds.), *Sexual behavior.* Boston: Little, Brown, 1972.

Brecher, E. *Treatment programs for sex offenders.* Washington, D.C.: National Institute of Law Enforcement Assistance Administration, 1977.

Brownmiller, S. *Against our will: Men, women, and rape.* New York: Simon & Schuster, 1975.

DeFrancis, V. *Protecting the child victim of sex crimes committed by adults.* Denver: American Humane Association, Children's Division, 1969.

Gebhard, P., Gagnon, J., Pomeroy, W., & Christenson, C. *Sex offenders: An analysis of types.* New York: Harper & Row, 1965.

Giarretto, H. The treatment of father-daughter incest: A psychosocial approach. *Children Today,* 1976, *5*(4), 2–5.

Groth, N., Burgess, A., & Holmstrom, L. Rape: Power, anger, and sexuality. *American Journal of Psychiatry,* 1977, *134*, 1239–1243.

Henn, F., Herjanic, M., & Vanderpearl, R. Forensic psychiatry: Profiles of two types of sex offenders. *American Journal of Psychiatry,* 1976, *133*, 694–696.

Marshall, W. The modification of sexual fantasies: A combined treatment approach to the reduction of deviant sexual behavior. *Behavior Research and Therapy,* 1973, *11*, 557–564.

McDonald, J. *Rape-offenders and their victims.* Springfield, Ill.: Charles Thomas, 1974.

Mohr, J., Turner, R., & Jerry, M. *Pedophilia and exhibitionism.* Toronto: University of Toronto Press, 1964.

Money, J. The therapeutic use of androgen-depleting hormone. *The Journal of Sex Research,* 1970, *6*, 165–173.

Oates, W. Religious attitudes and pastoral counseling. In H. Resnik & M. Wolfgang (Eds.), *Sexual Behavior.* Boston: Little, Brown, 1972.

Pacht, A. The rapist in treatment: Professional myths and psychological realities. In M. Walker & S. Brodsky (Eds.), *Sexual assualt.* Lexington, Mass: D.C. Health, 1976.

Pacht, A., & Cowden, J. An exploratory study of five hundred sex offenders. *Criminal Justice and Behavior*, 1974, *1*, 13–20.

Salzman, L. The psychodynamic approach to sex deviation. In H. Resnik & M. Wolfgang (Eds.), *Sexual behavior*. Boston: Little, Brown, 1972.

Stockton, M., Legum, L., & McAnaney, M. *A comprehensive treatment program for sex offenders*. Paper presented at the Convention of the Southeastern Psychological Association, Atlanta: March 1978.

Stürup, G. *Treatment of sexual offenders in Herstedvester, Denmark: The rapist*. Copenhagen: Munsgaard, 1968.

Secondary Impotence: Understanding, Prevention, and Treatment

BARRY W. MCCARTHY
American University

The myth of the male machine maintains that a "real man" should be ready and willing to have sex with any woman, any time, and in any situation. However, by age 40 over 90% of males will have at least one experience where they are unable to gain or maintain an erection sufficient for intercourse. Even more important, this myth causes males to be viewed as performance machines rather than as people. Trying to live up to these unrealistic performance demands is the major cause of male erectile difficulties (McCarthy, 1977b).

The word "potency" is an unfortunate, value-laden term. It connotes a range of powerful, self-assured masculine attitudes and behaviors. The term "impotence" refers not only to erectile problems, but also is a derogatory term connoting weakness and inadequacy. This points up one of the major psychological traps afflicting males, an overemphasis on sexual prowess defining their sense of self-esteem. A better terminology would be "erectile difficulties" which describes the sexual problem without excess meaning. However, since "impotence" is still so widely used both professionally and by the lay public, I will use it interchangeably with "erectile difficulties."

This paper will focus on secondary erectile problems, rather than primary impotence. Primary impotence means that the male has never had a successful intercourse experience with a woman. The majority of primary impotent males are able to masturbate to orgasm and many are orgasmic with a partner using manual or oral stimulation. Secondary impotence refers to a male who has had at least one successful intercourse (usually many satisfying intercourse experiences), but now has difficulty obtaining or maintaining an erection on a substantial percentage of occasions (25% or more).

I will use the P-LI-SS-IT model developed by Annon (1974) to provide a perspective for understanding and intervening with erectile problems. The P-LI-SS-IT model discusses four levels of intervention (permission giving, limited information, specific suggestions, and intensive sex therapy). This model can be used to conceptualize stages of sex counseling, done either individually, in a group, or workshop format with clients. For example, the first one or two sessions might focus more on permission giving and limited information. Subsequent sessions would continue to reinforce permission and information while supplementing this with specific, individualized sexual suggestions. Since all helping relationships would ideally include permission giving and information about sexuality we are all potentially sex counselors.

PERMISSION GIVING

A prime element is the counselor's encouraging a more pleasure-oriented and humanistic view of male sexuality rather than the performance-oriented, machine model. Rather than the male being expected to perform "at any time, with any woman, in any situation," the client could be helped to accept sexuality as an expression of himself as a person. The male is much more likely to be sexually functional if he has a feeling of choice and can comfortably make sexual requests. The male who feels demanded upon by the woman, that he'd better have a usable erection as soon as she's ready for intercourse, is practically setting himself up for erectile failure. The counselor can help the male see how self-defeating this attitude is and help him replace this by approaching the sexual experience with the expectation of mutual pleasure. The male needs to be aware of sexual turn-ons for himself, feel free to communicate his feelings and to make sexual requests. Rather than considering "foreplay" as a period where it is his "job" to turn the woman on and get her ready for intercourse, he can learn to be aware that this "pleasuring" period can be enjoyable and arousing for him also. The male's acceptance of the "give to get" principle ensures the woman's growing arousal is a turn-on for him, rather than a threat or a demand for performance. Intercourse becomes a natural extension of the pleasuring; in fact, intercourse might best be thought of as another pleasuring technique.

Equally important in the permission-giving phase is the permission to say "no." In the male's premarital socialization process, he is almost always the sexual initiator, pushing the woman (sometimes aggressively and inappropriately) to say "yes." It is almost unheard of for the male to say "no." This doublestandard approach to sexuality is bad enough premaritally, but even more harmful are its effects on adult sexual relationships. The counselor can support the concept that the male can feel free to say no to a sexual invitation without feeling in any way less masculine. He might say he's just not interested in sex at that particular time or he might prefer "to do" the woman either manually or orally, or he might prefer to simply engage in nondemand pleasuring. The counselor can make the male and/or couple aware of and comfortable with a range of alternative sexual experiences.

Permission to accept occasional inability to get or maintain an erection as being normal and natural rather than as a sign of "sexual failure" is an integral part of healthy male sexuality. Typically, males are not truthful about themselves sexually. For example, approximately one in five males have an unsuccessful first intercourse, either because of inability to get or maintain an erection or ejaculating before the penis enters the vagina. However, males do not admit this "failure" to friends, and thus the male feels that his was an extremely unusual and extremely humiliating experience. The same phenomenon occurs with occasional potency difficulties: although 90% of males have erectile difficulties, they are very seldom admitted. The notion that the male should always be able to respond sexually and perform intercourse is perfectionistic and clearly irrational. The counselor can not only provide the male with this information; the counselor can also encourage the male to honestly and frankly discuss experiences and concerns with friends.

LIMITED INFORMATION

The second level of intervention is limited information. Although over the last decade there has been a tremendous increase in information regarding human sexuality, it is striking that most of the media coverage and most of the books have focused on female sexuality (Barbach, 1975; Heiman, LoPiccolo, & LoPiccolo, 1976). This is especially tragic since some of the most interesting findings concern the aging male—with aging there is not a physiological need to ejaculate at each sexual opportunity and the male needs more direct penile stimulation to obtain erections (Butler & Lewis, 1975). Many of the basic facts of male sexual arousal such as the normal physiological process of waxing and waning of erections with prolonged pleasuring are not known to most males. To help provide this information a basic fact sheet on arousal and potency has been developed and is routinely distributed to students in human sexuality classes and clients.

Arousal and Erection Guidelines

1. By age 40, 90% of males experience at least one erectile failure; this is a normal occurrence, not be overreacted to as a sign of a major sex problem.

2. The great majority of potency problems are caused by psychological or relationship factors not medical or physiological malfunctions. To check out possible medical causes you could consult a urologist.

3. Erectile problems can be caused by a wide variety of factors including drinking too much, anxiety, depression, anger, frustration, fatigue, and just not feeling very aroused at that time or by that partner.

4. The key element is to accept the erectile difficulty as a situational problem, not to overreact and label yourself "impotent" or put yourself down as being a "failure" as a man.

5. There is a tendency for men to adopt the myth of the "male machine," ready to have an erection and intercourse at any time, with any woman, in any situation. You and your penis are human, not a performance machine.

6. One of the most pervasive myths is that if a man loses his initial erection, that means he's sexually turned off and must work to regain it. In reality, it is a natural physiological process for erections to wax and wane during a prolonged pleasuring period.

7. In a typical 45-minute pleasuring session before intercourse, the male's erection will wax and wane an average of three times. Subsequent erections are usually firmer and the ensuing orgasm more pleasurable.

8. You don't need an erect penis to satisfy a woman. Orgasms achieved through manual or oral stimulation are just as sexually satisfying. If you do have problems getting or maintaining an erection, the worse thing you can do is to stop the sexual interaction and put yourself down. Many women find it arousing to have the penis (erect or flaccid) used to stimulate the clitoral shaft or labia minora (inner lips).

9. A key element is to actively involve yourself in the pleasurable and sexually arousing interaction. An erection is a natural result of sexual arousal.

10. You cannot will or work at getting an erection. The worst thing you can do to yourself is to passively take a "spectator" role and observe the state of your penis. Sex requires active involvement. It is not a spectator sport.

11. It makes most sense for the woman to both initiate the moment of intercourse, and for her to guide your penis into her vagina. It takes pressure off you, and since the woman is the expert on her own sexuality, it is the most practical procedure.

12. You can learn to feel comfortable saying to your partner something like "I want the sex and pleasuring to go at a pace I'm comfortable with. When I feel pressure to perform sexually, I get uptight and sex is less good for you and me. Let's make it enjoyable for us by taking it at a comfortable pace."

13. Erectile problems do not affect the ability to ejaculate. Thus, many males learn to ejaculate with flaccid or semi-flaccid penises. The

male can again learn to ejaculate to an erect penis rather than a flaccid one.

14. One way to learn to feel comfortable with potency is through masturbation experiences. During masturbation you could practice gaining and losing erections, relearn to ejaculate to the cue of an erect penis, and focus on cues and fantasies which can be carried over to partner sex.

15. Morning erections should not generally be used for intercourse initiations. The morning erection can be a sign of arousal because of dreaming or because of being close to your partner, on the other hand it can be caused by a need to urinate. Too many men try to use their morning erections before they lose them. Remember, arousal and erections are regainable.

16. An important component in learning to feel comfortable with arousal and potency is to make clear, direct, assertive requests (not demands) of your partner for the type of sexual stimulation you find most arousing. It is important to learn to verbally and non-verbally guide your partner in how to pleasure and arouse you.

17. Stimulating a totally flaccid penis is usually counterproductive for sexual arousal. The male simply becomes more aware of the state of his penis. Instead you could engage in sensuous, non-genital, non-demand stimulation until there is some initial arousal and erection. The male can just lay back and enjoy this stimulation rather than trying to "will an erection."

18. Your attitude and self-thoughts can very much influence your arousal. We suggest that the key self-thought is that "sex and pleasure" go together not "sex and performance."

19. In thinking about a particular sexual experience, your feelings about it are best measured by your sense of pleasure and satisfaction rather than whether you got an erection, how hard it was, whether your partner was orgasmic. Accept that some sexual experiences will be great for both you and your partner, some will be better for one than the other, some will be mediocre, and there will be some which are poor. Do not put your sexual self-esteem on the line each time you have sex with a woman.

20. It is interesting to know that when you are sleeping, you get an erection every 90 minutes—4 or 5 erections a night. Sex and arousal are natural physiological functions. Don't block it by performance anxiety or putting yourself down. Give yourself (and your partner) permission to enjoy the pleasure of sexuality.

One function of the psychologist as an educator is to provide basic information about sexuality. I have been teaching a college course in human sexual behavior for several years and have been struck that the female/male ratio of students is approximately 3 to 1. Other possible educational formats include non-credit workshops on male/female sexuality and presentations on specific topics such as sexual dysfunctions, contraception, or changing sex roles. A student-written sex pamphlet (*Sex Facts for the A.U. Student, Second Edition*) has given credence to the notion that sex information is equally important for males and females. I believe that other universities and community agencies might find that it is worthwhile for a group of students or community people to write a sex pamphlet which includes a section of local resources and referrals.

In his/her role as educator, the counseling psychologist needs to make a special point of giving clear information about similarities and differences in male and female sexual response. Female sexual response is more complex (not better or worse, just more complex) than male sexual response. The woman may be non-orgasmic, singly orgasmic, or multi-orgasmic and this could occur during pleasuring/foreplay, intercourse, or afterplay/afterglow. The male has to understand and accept this rather than demanding the woman have a simultaneous orgasm, or be multi-orgasmic, or have a single orgasm which must occur during intercourse.

SPECIFIC SEXUAL SUGGESTIONS

The third level of intervention is specific sexual suggestions. This usually occurs in the context of short-term counseling or in sexuality workshops. Suggestions include (1) helping the male to feel comfortable saying to his partner "I like you and I enjoy our affectionate relationship. I want to become more sexually involved, but I want to go at my own pace. When I feel I have to perform sexually, I get uptight and that makes sex less pleasurable for you and for me. Let's go at a comfortable pace and make sex enjoyable for both of us." This seemingly straightforward assertive statement is a direct reversal of the male role of not sharing feelings or admitting weakness and often requires a good deal of behavioral rehearsal with the client.

(2) The male can use masturbation and/or practice with a partner to get an erection, then stop stimulation until the erection wanes, and then engage in stimulation and obtain a second erection. Learning that an erection can be regained is crucial in feeling secure with the arousal process.

(3) The woman can initiate and guide intromission. This serves to reduce anticipatory anxiety and pressure on the man to skillfully insert. The woman is the expert on her vagina and she is often more comfortable and adept at intromission than the male. This also serves to make her a more active partner in the sexual interaction.

(4) Put a temporary (perhaps a week or two) ban on intercourse, but not on sex. The couple is encouraged to actively engage in nongenital and genital pleasuring. With the pressure for intercourse removed, the male

often finds his arousal and erections much stronger. He learns he can sexually satisfy his partner with his hands and/or tongue quite effectively. He can learn to feel comfortable being orgasmic with his partner's manual or oral stimulation.

(5) Reduce anxiety about sexual performance. There are a variety of strategies and techniques including relaxation training, guided imagery, use of fantasy, expressing anxious feelings to your partner, actively reinvolving yourself in pleasuring your partner, etc. (McCarthy, 1977a).

(6) The male is encouraged to continue masturbating, and to relearn to be orgasmic to an erect penis. Many men with erectile difficulties continue to be orgasmic with a partner or through masturbation, but more and more with semiflaccid or totally flaccid penises. Remember, arousal/erection and orgasm/ejaculation are two separate functions, seldom are both impaired. It is reinforcing for the man to relearn he can ejaculate to the cue of an erect penis during masturbation and gives hope that he can do this with a partner.

These three levels of intervention can also be used in preventive programs. These concepts could be made more readily available through means such as a course, pamphlet, and workshops on human sexuality.

SEX THERAPY

The fourth level of intervention—sex therapy—includes elements of permission-giving, limited information, and specific suggestions. Additional components of sex therapy include taking a detailed sex history, providing consultation on a weekly basis, individualizing a program of sexual exercises, and focusing on individual and relationship issues. The couple are seen conjointly with the sexual relationship viewed as the client. It is considerably more difficult to treat males without partners, although an individualized program focusing on desensitization, behavioral rehearsal, and cognitive restructuring can be utilized. In general, it is recommended that a male therapist treat a single male.

Secondary impotence is one of the more difficult sexual dysfunctions to treat. According to Masters and Johnson (1970), it has a 10% recidivism rate, which is one of the highest. The more chronic and pervasive the erectile problem and the more it is tied into the couple's dysfunctional system, the more difficult it is to treat successfully. However, even with this caution, success rates are over 60% and as high as 80% (Masters & Johnson, 1970; Kaplan, 1974; McCarthy, Ryan, & Johnson, 1975).

Central to the treatment of secondary impotence is the involvement of both partners, enjoying the sexual experience for the pleasure it brings rather than evaluating it as good or bad depending on the state of the penis: It is best if the male can actively involve himself in the sexual interaction rather than be a spectator; if the woman can be supportive and enjoy her sexuality rather than be condescending or demanding; and if the couple has a continuing commitment to communicate, experiment, and share. An important ingredient of the sex therapy process is for the couple to deal with disappointments and frustrations that invariably occur when learning a new manner of relating sexually. Sex therapy is helpful in facilitating the attitude that a couple's sex life is capable of growing and developing if they maintain their commitment to nondemand pleasuring and to communication.

The sex therapy model is based on cases where there is no major organic, individual, or couple problem. The therapist needs to be aware of these factors in modifying his treatment approach or making referrals. There have recently been breakthroughs in assessing and treating organic factors. There is a penile tumescence monitoring device which records erections during sleep to determine whether the erectile difficulty is primarily organic or psychological (Fisher, 1975). For organic impotence a newly developed penile implant procedure is an alternative (Scott, Bradley, & Timm, 1973). In some cases, testosterone replacement therapy is a crucial adjunctive technique. Where organic issues are important, consultation between the urologist and therapist is vital. Where major psychological problems are evident, individual psychotherapy, either in conjunction with or instead of sex therapy, is advisable. This same principle applies to marital problems; marriage counseling can be adjunctive to or the treatment of choice instead of sex therapy. Of course, it is possible to integrate marital therapy and sex therapy (Messersmith, 1976).

In summary, erectile difficulties (secondary impotence) is problematic for many males. Much of the reason lies in unrealistic expectations of male sexual performance. A lack of understanding of sexual arousal and erectile function, a performance-oriented rather than pleasure-oriented view of sexuality, and a reluctance to communicate with one's partner about their sexual experience all contribute to the difficulty. At a societal level, male and female sexual behaviors and feelings are in a process of change. Erectile difficulties often are a sign that the process of adjustment to these changes has not been successful. My hope is that the strategies and techniques presented in this paper will facilitate understanding, prevention, and treatment of erectile problems.

REFERENCES

Annon, J. *The behavioral treatment of sexual problems: Brief therapy.* Honolulu: Kapiolani Health Services, 1974.

Barbach, L. *For yourself: The fulfillment of female sexuality.* Garden City, New York: Doubleday, 1975.

Butler, R., & Lewis, M. *Sex after sixty.* New York: Harper & Row, 1975.

Fisher, C. The assessment of nocturnal REM erection in the differential diagnosis of sexual impotence. *Journal of Sex and Marital Therapy,* 1975, *1*, 277–289.

Heiman, J., LoPiccolo, L., & LoPiccolo, J. *Becoming orgasmic: A sexual growth program for women.* Englewood Cliffs, N.J.: Prentice-Hall. 1976.

Kaplan, H. *The new sex therapy.* New Yourk: Brunner/Mazel, 1974.

Masters, W., & Johnson, V. *Human sexual inadequacy.* Boston: Little, Brown, 1970.

McCarthy, B. Strategies and techniques for the reduction of sexual anxiety. *Journal of Sex and Marital Therapy,* 1977, *3*(4), 243–248. (a)

McCarthy, B. *What you still don't know about male sexuality.* New York: Crowell, 1977. (b)

McCarthy, B., Ryan, M., & Johnson, F. *Sexual awareness: A practical approach.* San Francisco: Boyd & Fraser, 1975.

Messersmith, C. Sex therapy and the marital system. In D. Olson (Ed.), *Treating relationships.* Lake Mills, Ia.: Graphic Publishing, 1976.

Scott, F., Bradley, W., & Timm, G. Management of erectile impotence: Use of implantable inflatable prosthesis. *Urology,* 1973, *2*, 80–82.

Divided Allegiance:
Men, Work, and Family Life

MICHAEL BERGER AND LARRY WRIGHT
Georgia State University

> In the sweat of thy face shalt thou eat bread till thou return unto the ground, for out of it thou was taken; for dust thou art and unto dust thou shalt return [Genesis 3, 19].

The sin for which the Lord expelled Adam from the Garden was that of heeding the voice of his wife rather than the injunction of the Lord. Adam followed the logic and the loyalties of his private world. And his punishment was to be thrust into the public world, the world of work, a world which was now to be separate and alien from the private world. "So he drove out the man and he placed at the east of Eden cherubims and a flaming sword. . . . "

As Marx noted, for centuries this alienated world has been the primary world for men. In the past 100 years, due to the ability of industrialized nations to provide sufficient goods so that adults need not work full-time to survive, men have become more aware of other options for themselves, other parts of themselves. Now, like the image of the soul in Plato's *The Symposium,* the sundered halves of the once-whole human being are pursuing each other across the great waste of the world.[1]

Our culture socializes men to view work in a stereotypical and sexist way. We teach children that men must work. We teach male children that a man's identity as a person is based on whether he works and how well he does his work (competence usually being measured by earnings or status). For males in our society, work is primary. All other roles are secondary. At most, a male's family responsibilities consist of being a provider and of helping, occasionally, with the children. All other family responsibilities

Note: The authors are professionals. As such, we subscribe to the dominant cultural belief that having a "career" is good. We emphatically do not recommend this value for everyone.

The contribution of Stephen Berger in a) keeping the senior author honest, and b) explicating the Genesis incident, is gratefully acknowledged.

[1]We are indebted to Sidney Monas for calling our attention to this image.

are "naturally" left to the wife. So, for men in our culture, there is a segregation of work and family responsibilities (Pleck, 1975).

The idea that men work and women run the home persists (Rapoport & Rapaport, 1977) even though the dual-employment marriage has become the modal family type (Pleck, in press). Individuals who wish to create and maintain a new type of marriage have been socialized into and measure themselves against traditional values. Clinicians tend to share these traditional values in their private lives and when doing marital or family therapy. While the women's movement has forced clinicians to take into account the new roles open to female clients, no equivalent movement has demanded that clinicians deal with new roles potentially available to men. It is time for clinicians to support male clients in examining roles other than the traditionally male ones. To do this, clinicians must be willing to recognize the importance of societal factors (such as the structure of work roles and settings) that affect the lives of clients. Men do not live only in an intrapsychic world. Moreover, clinicians must be willing to deal with the threat to their own life choices posed by the reality of a male client who is willing to give up the higher status traditional male values. We suspect it will be easier for clinicians to support a female client in espousing values seen as traditionally male than to support a male client in living in accord with values traditionally reserved for women.

THE WORK LIFE CYCLE OF MEN

According to adult life cycle theorists (for example, Erikson, 1950; D. Levinson, Darrow, Klein, M. Levinson, & McKee, 1973), if he is successful, a man's career follows a regular and predictable pattern.[2] In its ideal type, this cycle begins when a man chooses a career and ends with retirement. Principal influences on a man at the time of career choice are educational experiences, his drive to better himself, and the influence of the models of friends, peers, teachers, and so forth.

After a career is chosen and educational preparations completed, the next stage of the work life cycle is the stage during which a man must learn to "play the game," must learn the unwritten as well as the written rules for success. This is likely to be a workaholic stage because it is during this period that men are expected to make their impression on their superiors, even if it takes 80 hours a week to do so. Males during this stage are likely to be absent family members.

Another factor that often has profound effects on the family is the mobility required of men during this stage of their careers. Part of the necessary attitudes that accompany getting ahead require that the man move often and move his family with him if he is to "make it." Such

---

[2]Needless to say, these formulations, like all typologies, simplify the world they describe.

behavior requires that other family members subordinate their goals to the husband's career demands.

The next predictable stage in the work life cycle is the "failure" stage. *Every man fails in his career.* No man accomplishes all he wanted to accomplish, could have accomplished, or should have accomplished. Regardless of how much has been achieved during his career, it isn't enough, and this failure is felt as due to personal shortcomings rather than to institutional constraints or societal factors. This stage of the cycle coincides with what Levinson et al. (1973) refer to as the mid-life crisis.

The mid-life crisis is a family crisis as well as an individual trauma. The male, having failed to conquer and dominate the work world now turns inward to seek solace, satisfaction, and meaning from his marriage and his family. Chronologically, this usually occurs when the children have left or are in the process of leaving and the wife, having spent years looking inward to the family and the marriage, is now beginning to look outside the home for her satisfactions. Thus, the timing of spouse's developmental needs is not in synchrony (Levinson et al.,1973). Couples find themselves passing in the night.

The next predictable stage in a man's work life cycle occurs when he retires. This stage can be a time of great stress for both spouses. For man has lost the realm which has been his principal identity since early adulthood—his "occupation is gone." He is now a being without a function. He may become a sort of supernumerary at home, "underfoot" because his wife has spent the previous years with total responsibility for the home. He may seek reassurance and attention from his spouse in an almost child-like manner. Many men experience a strong feeling of purposelessness and loss during the early days of this stage of the work life cycle; indeed, many men behave as if the task during this stage was to prepare to die (Bernard, 1973; Duvall, 1971).

Men who are not successful in the usual cultural terms do not possess anything so grandiose as a career. Typically, they end their work lives in the same kinds of jobs and settings in which they began them. For such men, relocation and social or physical mobility are not reality issues though they may figure in nightmares as indices of success by which the individual judges himself to have failed. Still, for such men, the scheduling and structure of work (for example, a predictable shift, mandatory overtime, and so forth) demands accommodation on the part of other family members.

ALTERNATIVE WORK-CAREER PATTERNS

The bleak picture painted above is not given in the nature of the world; rather it is the product of a particular societal organization. However, our society is changing, even if slowly, and alternative patterns of integrating work and family careers are becoming available (although not socially approved) for men. As pointed out above, in most families today the man is not the sole bread-winner. The number of wives who work at least part-time passed the fifty percent mark in the early 1970s (Hoffman, 1976), and the patterns of integration of work and family responsibilities are in the process of changing for both men and women.

The Rapoports (1977) have described at length the dual-career marriage in which both spouses are engaged in full-time careers requiring a great deal of commitment. Adopting this style of marriage is likely to require both spouses to rethink their priorities and objectives in marriage. The dual-career couple has no wife to perform on a full-time basis the myriad tasks of housekeeping and childcare. Therefore, the husband is likely to become more involved in areas that have traditionally been viewed as "women's work."

Wright and Berger (Reference Note 3) have reviewed studies dealing with dual-employment families and have suggested that roles for men must change. Men need to assume more responsibility for housework and childcare if wives are to be able to devote themselves to their work.

Other alternative roles for men include part-time employment either as a style in itself or as part of being a house-husband (Levine, 1976). The house-husband role is clearly more deviant than simply becoming more involved in household responsibilities, but this role may be the most intelligent course in many families. If the wife is better prepared for work educationally, psychologically, and experientially than the husband, and if the husband prefers to remain at home caring for the house and children, then this should be a socially viable alternative for the couple. Yet it is clear that such a marital arrangement would be the object of a great deal of negative social sanction. It therefore takes a courageous couple to embark on such a course. Men will have to deal with socialization that suggests "woman's work" is emasculating. Women will need to abandon their scripting and tolerate the reality that some husbands may take better care of children than some wives.

The alternative styles of integrating work and family roles, briefly outlined above, certainly offer men opportunities for structuring their lives in non-traditional ways and avoid some of the pitfalls of the traditional work life cycle. Most of the constraints that men espousing alternative roles will experience grow directly out of psychosocial lag—that is, cultures persist in supporting values and role models long after the societal structures based on such values have changed. A man is judged by traditional guidelines as to what a man should be. A man who deviates from these guidelines will be devalued and will experience strong pressures from his peers to "act like a man" (Bear & Berger, Reference Note 1).

Another powerful constraining influence on men who attempt to adopt alternate values in integrating work and family life, comes from what the Rapoports (1977) refer to as role-cycling dilemmas. Role-cycling dilemmas are the result of irreconcilable demands of work and family. For example, the child-bearing years are a time of frantic demands for child care (which in this culture is expected to be provided by a family member at home whether this is desirable or not) and are also years in which a very high degree of strain is placed on a young family's financial resources. So the demand for both spouses to work and generate income will be very high, while the demand for both spouses to be available to the children will also be great.

Additional constraints regarding nontraditional roles for men derive from the ways in which the nature and structure of work is institutionally defined. For men who are trying to "make it" at work, the rules are clear: the job comes first and family second. Men are expected to work long hours, to travel, to relocate, to attend social functions, and in general to arrange their lives around the requirements of their job—not around the requirements of their spouse or family. The need to remain promotable creates a nightmare of conflicting pressures for the man who wants to "make it" *both* at home and at work. Rosen and his associates (Rosen & Jerdee, 1973, 1974; Rosen, Jerdee, & Prestwich, 1975) have demonstrated how men are expected by their companies to display consistently sex-stereotyped behaviors if they wish to be successful in their careers. Kantor (1977) has recently confirmed this for both men and women.

Taking all this into account, it is not surprising that men who try to live nontraditionally both at home and at work put themselves into a number of stressful situations. Moreover, nontraditional marriages are stressful for women as well as men. It is difficult to be comfortable as a "stranger in a strange land," and until the societal constraints which support traditional marriages alter, couples living untraditionally will lack acceptance. Lacking acceptance, they will find it difficult to accept themselves and their marital choices. Sadly, then, most couples will attribute their marital difficulties to their own personal shortcomings rather than to the cultural and institutional constraints that may well be the greatest source of their discomfort (Berger, Foster, Wallston, & Wright, 1977).

CLINICAL IMPLICATIONS

Couples espousing nontraditional life styles will have nontraditional problems. As Stachkowik (Reference Note 2) has noted, all families have a right to a therapist who likes them. Families espousing nontraditional life styles deserve a therapist who can tolerate nontraditional ways of thinking about marriage and family life, and who is able to facilitate innovative solutions.

The first step in working with a client in a nontraditional marriage should be to help the client clarify his/her values concerning the roles of husband, wife, father, mother, and so forth, in the kind of family they have chosen to create. It will probably also be necessary to assist the client in challenging early assumptions about what men and women "do" and about what it means to assume familial roles. Values will need to be challenged and priorities reassessed and reordered.

Clinicians may also have to spend a good deal of time in supporting the deviant roles that their clients have chosen. The lack of support that the client has experienced in his/her world for the role he/she is living is likely to be a major factor in bringing them into therapy. Another service the therapist could provide men involved in nontraditional marriages is the development of consciousness-raising groups for men. These groups could provide an effective forum for questioning the sex-role stereotypes learned in early life and reinforced by the culture. The emphasis here would be to allow men the freedom to develop into the kind of people they would like to be. Men (and women) need not be restricted by social stereotypes of what they can or should *be* or how they should live their lives.

Finally, it should be noted that, for men to change their roles, changes must occur in the realm of institutional policies. As men change and insist on their right to define themselves in nontraditional ways, institutions will be forced to follow. But institutions change slowly, old values die hard, and we need support during the interim. Therapists, therefore, must learn to help men to support one another in changing these institutional practices and in living lives now that are in accordance with their desires. It is not enough to deal with the version of the world internalized in clients' heads. The time has come to change the world outside the client.

CONCLUSION

As marriage and men's roles in marriage and in the family change, some men will seek to define themselves in new and different ways. How successful they will be in these attempts will be determined by the amount of support they receive and by the degree to which institutional constraints can be overcome. As clinicians, we may be exacerbating the problems of our clients who are attempting to change. We grew up in this culture and we benefit from it. We are not immune to the same influences, values and socialization processes that create problems for our clients. Therefore, we have a responsibility to reexamine our own values, assumptions, and expectations regarding the "appropriate" roles that men can play in both work and family spheres. We must not accept the limits that the culture has prescribed as "natural" or even appropriate. As C. Wright Mills wrote just before his death, social change is necessary when "most men perceive their lives as a series of traps . . . and personal problems are public issues" (1959, p. 1).

REFERENCE NOTES

1. Bear, S. & Berger, M. Even cowboys sing the blues: Difficulties experienced by men espousing untraditional life styles. Submitted to *Sex Roles: A journal of research.*

2. Stachkowick, J. Personal communication to senior author, 1974.
3. Wright, L., & Berger, M. Dual-employment families and the family life cycle. Submitted to *The Family Coordinator*.

REFERENCES

Berger, M., Foster, M., Wallston, B., & Wright, L. You and me against the world: Dual-career couples and joint job seeking. *Journal of Research and Development in Education*, 1977, *10*, 30–37.

Bernard, J. *The future of marriage*. New York: Bantam Books, 1973.

Duvall, E. *Family development* (4th ed). Philadelphia: Lippincott, 1971.

Erikson, E. *Childhood and society*. New York: Norton, 1950.

Hoffman, L. *Change in family roles, socialization, and sex differences*. Paper presented at the Annual Meeting of the National Council on Family Relations, October, 1976.

Kantor, R. *Men and women of the corporation*. New York: Basic Books, 1977.

Levine, J. *Men who care for children*. Philadelphia: Lippincott, 1976.

Levinson, D., Darrow, C., Klein, E., Levinson, M., & McKee, B. The psychosocial development of men in early adulthood and the mid-life crisis. In D. Ricks, A. Thomas, & M. Roff (Eds.), *Life history research in psychopathology* (Vol.3). Minneapolis: University of Minnesota Press, 1973.

Mills, C. *The sociological imagination*. New York: Oxford Press, 1959.

Pleck, J. *Work and family roles: From sex-patterned segregation to integration*. Paper presented at the Annual Meeting of the American Sociological Association, San Francisco, 1975.

Pleck, J. Men's new roles in the family: Housework and child care. In C. Safilios-Rothschild (Ed.), *Family and sex roles*, in press.

Rapoport, R., & Rapoport, R. *Dual-career families reexamined: New integrations of work and family*. New York: Harper & Row, 1977.

Rosen. B., & Jerdee, T. The influence of sex-role stereotyping on evaluations of male and female supervisory behavior. *Journal of Applied Psychology*, 1973, *57*, 44–48.

Rosen, B., & Jerdee, T. Sex stereotyping in the executive suite. *Harvard Business Review*, 1974, *52*, 45–48.

Rosen, B., Jerdee, T., & Prestwich, T. Dual-career marital adjustment: Potential effects of discriminatory managerial attitudes. *Journal of Marriage and the Family*, 1975, *37*, 565–572.

Facilitating the Birth Process and Father-Child Bonding

JEAN GEARING
Planned Parenthood
Gainesville, Florida

A major re-evaluation of the role of the father is presently underway among growing numbers of social scientists and parents. Many cultural changes occurring during this late 20th century period are radically altering the structure of American family networks. The rising divorce rate and the tremendous increase in single-parent families, which are frequently father-absent families, have prompted research interest in the deleterious effects of father absence upon children. Child abuse is another problem area of father-child interaction that has drawn professional concern. Another major area of change has been in popular conceptions of appropriate sex roles, especially women's roles, because of the influence of the women's liberation movement. Effective contraception has freed women from the necessity of remaining at home most of their lives rearing children. Instead, more women are working full-time while demanding a more egalitarian division of responsibilities for house and child care (Bernard, 1972).

The combination of concern over pathological father/child interactions, demands from feminist theorists for the restructuring of sex roles, and the growing realization that little was actually known about the norms of fathering has led in the past three years to a growing amount of research into paternal behavior in whole families. One surprising discovery has been the strong interest fathers express in their infants and a willingness to share in caretaking activities. The common cultural myth that American men are not interested in their children until they are walking and talking has been disproved in studies by Parke, O'Leary, and West, (1972); Parke and O'Leary (1976); Rendina and Dickerscheid (1976); and Fein (1976). In another study, McIntire, Nass, and Battistone (1974) surveyed the attitudes of unmarried college-age men toward parenting and found that 90% of the men agreed with statements that fathers should participate in infant care. Studies of actual caretaking behavior, such as Kotelchuck (1972), have not reported such high percentages of childcare sharing, perhaps due to the fact that couples were following traditional division of labor patterns. Typically, in most studies of father/mother/infant interaction, the mothers spend more time engaged in routine caretaking activities, whereas the fathers spend more time engaged in visually attending to, holding, or in stimulating play with their babies. Kotelchuck (1976), describing a series of experiments examining infants' separation protest, reported that in stress situations, mothers were slightly preferred by most infants over fathers, but in nonstress situations most infants were as strongly attached to their fathers as they were to their mothers. In America today, most middle-class men want to participate in fathering from the time their babies are born, and they have become significant, salient others to their infants by one year of age.

Another phenomenon occurring in the past ten years which indicates men's strong interest in fathering, has been the incredible growth in the numbers of men participating in prepared childbirth classes during pregnancy and being present during labor and the birth of their children. Although many men no doubt enroll in classes primarily to learn how to support their wives during labor, most men react extremely positively when they become actual participants in the birth process. In Tanzer's study (1967) of prepared versus conventional childbirth, the husbands who had been present during the birth of their children repeatedly offered to describe the personal impact the experience had had on them. Greenberg and Morris (1974), in their clinical study of the reactions of new fathers, reported that the men experienced a feeling of elation or "high" and an increased sense of self-esteem, as well as a strong attraction toward the newborn, when they witnessed the birth.

In sum, fathers appear to be capable of nurturant behavior toward their infants and are strongly interested in them, although they engage in less caretaking and more play with their infants than mothers. Fathers who may decide to participate in the birth process to aid their wives also derive great personal satisfaction from doing so. The traditional, noninvolved "breadwinner" image of the father is changing into a new, more actively involved father, who is willing to assume some caretaking responsibility for his children soon after birth.

Despite the fact that young men are interested in becoming involved fathers, many factors remain that interfere with an easy transition to an involved style of fathering. The effect of major social changes and new role options has also meant an increase in ambivalence towards having children and establishing nuclear families. The combination of greater affluence, better education, increased mobility, the threat of overpopulation, and urban isolation has reduced traditional social pressures on young people to marry and to have children. The popular ethic places an increasing emphasis on individual growth, perhaps at the expense of the development of a sense of responsibility for dependent others required in establishing a family. The negative effects of having children upon one's career, personal development, and even marital happiness have received much media attention in recent years, whereas the positive effects of childraising have been deemphasized. Psychologists do not even know what differences in personality development occur between those individuals who choose to have children and those who choose to remain childless, though the change from the childless to the childrearing state is surely one of the most radical lifestyle shifts a person can undertake.

The current generation of young adults was reared in mostly suburban, isolated nuclear families that stressed highly polarized stereotyped sex-role behavior. Individuals, both men and women, are rejecting these rigid patterns of masculinity and femininity in favor of new forms that stress the advantages of androgyny. These people who are attempting to restructure their attitudes and create different types of families for their children, are experiencing difficulties due to their own early cultural conditioning and the lack of positive social reinforcement. Men who are trying to become involved fathers are encountering many problems. The lack of successful role models, practical instruction and experience in childcare, and societal acknowledgment result in almost no socialization for the fathering role for the young male in our culture. Parenthood is a difficult transition to master at any time, but becoming a parent when the role itself is undergoing transition is even more problematic.

Professionals need to develop programs to aid individuals who are exploring alternative parental roles. A strong emphasis should be placed on the importance of the fathering role, especially its positive and negative effects on the man as well as on the child within the interactional system of the family. Although certainly not comprising the majority of young parents, many college-educated young people express a desire to alter the traditional allocation of financial and childrearing responsibilities within their families. These individuals are voluntary participants in a social experiment of unprecedented extent. It is imperative that programs be developed to facilitate this process of self-induced change, even as researchers study the event.

One model for a counseling program for new parents is proposed in this paper. This program combines educational and counseling techniques designed to ease men's transition to parenthood in a three-stage program before, during, and after the birth of the first child. The intention of this effort is to develop men's innate potentials for nurturance and fathering, with an emphasis on accepting personal responsibility for parenting. Each participating man is viewed as one half of a dyad in transition to parenthood, with the woman partner included in some aspects of this program. The focus is on men because of their relative lack of socialization for an active parenting role.

Women are prepared for the assumption of motherhood by the changes occurring within their bodies. The expectant mother, as soon as she shows evidence of her pregnancy, is barraged externally with information and advice that helps to change her self-perceptions. Her identity expands into motherhood. American culture reinforces a pregnant woman much more actively than it does an expectant father, whom it scarcely acknowledges. Men have no physiological reminders of their changing roles. The husband is encouraged to be supportive and even indulgent toward his pregnant wife, while his own anxieties are underplayed. Colman and Colman (1971), in their book *Pregnancy: The Psychological Experience,* discuss some of the problems of the expectant father. These include increased financial worries; identification with or jealousy of the woman's ability to bear children; incest anxieties prompted by the new maternal role of the wife; unresolved sibling rivalries; remembrance of his own father and anxieties about being a father to his own child; the wife's increased physical and emotional dependency; possible sexual deprivation; fears about labor and delivery, especially if he plans to participate as a coach in a prepared birth; and the lifestyle changes necessary when the baby is born. Medical studies of expectant fathers reveal that more than one in ten will develop psychogenic physical symptoms, many of which mimic pregnancy and which disappear after the birth of the child (Trethowan & Conlon, 1965). This phenomenon has been labeled the *couvade syndrome,* by Trethowan, for the rituals undertaken by expectant fathers in primitive cultures during pregnancy and birth. Psychiatrists have reported an increase in psychological and behavioral complaints, and even psychoses, in some men during their wives' pregnancies or shortly after the birth of their children (Lacoursiere, 1972).

STAGE ONE OF THE COUNSELING PROGRAM:

The first stage of the counseling program is designed to help expectant fathers work through anxieties related to their wives' pregnancies and to help them develop a coherent fathering role. Men would enroll in this program approximately three months prior to the birth of their first child, at about the same time many couples begin prepared childbirth classes. Childbirth educators, although they encourage male participation in birth, of necessity focus on preparing women physically and psychologically for the birth process. Most childbirth educators are nurses, and although they are aware of expectant fathers' anxieties, they are not always trained in counseling. Nearly all are women and thus not capable of being good role models of fathering. Couples would be urged to enroll in some form of prepared childbirth training in addition to the counseling program offered to men interested in becoming involved fathers. The program stresses practical instruction in childcare, with real infants and both male and female adult role models in actual homelike situations. Demonstrations and discussion by already actively involved fathers would reinforce the expectant fathers' desire to participate in childcare by showing the novices that these tasks can be mastered through practice and require no uniquely feminine "maternal" instinct. The real-life situations enable the men to encounter men who have effectively mastered the transition to fatherhood without damaging their masculine identity. This potentially stress-free opportunity to learn and practice childcare skills with already successful male models should enable the expectant fathers to gain confidence in their abilities before they need to use them.

Group sessions for the expectant fathers without their partners present, led by male counselors experienced in fathering and familiar with the literature, are another major part of the first stage of the counseling program. The purpose of these sessions is to verbalize the men's feelings and attitudes toward fatherhood and the changes occurring in their lives. The range of fathering behavior, different fathering styles, and the importance of the fathering role, how it differs from and complements the mother's role, should all be stressed by the group leader. He may want to introduce actual research results or use literary sources as well as personal reminiscences to facilitate group process. An important area for work is the relationship each man had with his own father and how it influenced his conceptions of the role as he wants to enact it with his own child.

The final component of the first stage are couple sessions with each husband and wife led by teams of male and female counselors. Robert Fein (1976), in his study of 30 couples before and after they became parents, has found that one important factor easing men's adjustment to fatherhood is congruence with their wives on parental role dimensions. Congruence was more important than choosing any particular style. The counselors should stress mutual agreement but not insist on any one distribution pattern of childcare, household, or financial responsibilities. Another important function of these couple sessions is to work through problems occurring in the marital relationship during the pregnancy and those expected after the baby is born. One coping strategy is the development of plans that will enable husband and wife to continue spending some time alone with each other after the baby is born. Gilman and Knox (1976) found that husbands who re-established courtship behavior with their wives after the birth of the baby reported greater marital satisfaction. Marital satisfaction strongly influences satisfaction with parenting for both men and women (Russell, 1974).

STAGE TWO OF THE COUNSELING PROGRAM:

The second stage of the program involves the actual process of birth and the period immediately following, and requires cooperation from hospital personnel. Husbands are urged to remain with their wives during labor and delivery if it is possible, and the new family is given time alone after birth in a physically comfortable setting to become acquainted with each other. Klaus and Kennell (1976), in their book *Maternal-Infant Bonding,* stress the importance of the first hour after birth to the formation of the attachment bond between mother and infant. During this period the neonate is more active and alert than it will be during the next twenty-four hours, and eye-to-eye and skin-to-skin contact between mother and child in mutual exploration at this time creates long-lasting affectionate attachment bonds. Greenberg and Morris (1974) emphasize the importance of the newborn's innate reflex activity in eliciting an emotional response from new fathers. The intensity of this response, labelled "engrossment" by Greenberg and Morris, surprised the men, who prior to the birth had not expected to become so fascinated or personally involved with their babies. This response may be an equivalent of the mother/infant attachment bond. If this is so, the active hour after birth would also be a critical period for development of a paternal/infant attachment bond.

Rooming-in, with the father permitted to stay with the mother overnight, if both desire it, would be the ideal situation after birth in the hospital. Both parents could share childcare from the beginning, secure in the knowledge that trained professionals were available for assistance and relief. Mutually acceptable allocation of infant care could be established and shifted to the home when both parents were ready. An awkward split in the new family could be avoided, and both parents would be recognized as joint care-givers. Gollober (1976), commenting on the need for father/infant postpartal interaction, states that "family-centered" maternity care in most hospitals has actually remained mother-centered care. The new father is still routinely excluded from formal childcare teaching sessions conducted by the nursing staff, which hampers his learning about his infant. Gollober (1976) recommends giving the father opportunities to interact with his infant on all levels: distal, physical, and visual. The present program maximizes these opportunities when birth occurs in the hospital setting. Lind (1974) reports from Sweden that fathers who were taught and practiced childcare skills during the immediate postpartum period in the hospital were more involved with their infants at six months. This and other studies (Fein, 1976; Greenberg & Morris, 1974; Leonard, 1976; Parke & Sawin, 1976) support the contention that initial contact between father and infant has consequences for later caretaking behavior and should be facilitated by hospital personnel. Fathers will need full-time paternity leaves for at least one week to implement these suggestions.

STAGE THREE OF THE COUNSELING PROGRAM:

After the baby is born and the young family has returned home, the third stage of the counseling program begins. It consists of the continuation of the fathers' group sessions, meeting less frequently than before the birth. The new fathers can exchange birth experiences, share frustrations, and receive continued reinforcement for their contributions as involved fathers. Men from these groups could also serve as role models for other groups of expectant fathers.

Both parents should be encouraged to come to the baby's medical check-ups. Information on how to organize and run a baby-sitting cooperative with other young couples and a possible telephone hotline with older and more experienced parents would be two services that could be begun by professionals and maintained through the parents' efforts. Both of these serve as partial substitutes for the extended-family network.

BARRIERS TO INVOLVED FATHERHOOD

In order for fathers to participate more fully in childrearing, however, many institutional changes are necessary. The most important of these is for our society to recognize the benefits, to both parent and child, of active fathers who participate in their children's lives. Flexible work schedules, paternity leaves, and decently paid part-time jobs must be made available to parents when their children are young. Many more childcare centers located near or in the workplace should be created. Maternity centers that offer genuinely family-centered care in a home-like atmosphere while providing expert medical assistance before, during, and after birth could easily accommodate a program for expectant fathers similar to the one proposed in this paper. Maternity centers offer the advantages of home birth with the expert care of a hospital and can serve as a community center and information resource for young parents; unfortunately, few exist in the United States, although they are common in the Netherlands and Scandinavian countries. The growing trend toward home births is evidence that some alternative to traditional hospital methods of handling labor and delivery is desired by expectant parents (Ritchie & Swanson, 1976).

The American family is under severe stress, but many young parents are trying to establish more flexible and humanistic families that can adapt to the conditions of the modern world and not interfere with the self-development of any member. One of the most significant changes is men becoming actively involved in all aspects of their children's lives, especially caring for young infants. However, men receive little actual preparation for an active, participant fathering role. Mental health professionals can create counseling and educational programs that can offer a combination of information, practice in childcare skills, and counseling to aid men's transition to a new, more rewarding style of fathering. The possible benefits to both parents and their children are immeasurable; and to the extent that happier families are more stable and longer lasting, the possible benefits to society as a whole are also great. Much lipservice has been paid in modern America to strengthening the family, and many intervention programs have been designed and implemented to cope with families already in trouble. Unfortunately, few preventive programs designed to ease men's and women's transition to parenthood have been created. One such program is described by J. L. Resnick, M. B. Resnick, Packer, and Wilson (1978). It is the only program found in an extensive search of the literature that combines pre- and post-natal classes for parents and that emphasizes the role of the father. Many persons write of the need for programs for men (Heise, 1975; Hott, 1976; Gollober, 1976; Leonard, 1976). Obviously, more than one program is needed. It is sincerely hoped that this article will stimulate the further interest of professionals in the area of men's transition to fatherhood and the establishment of more programs.

REFERENCES

Bernard, J. *The future of marriage*. New York: World Publishing Company, 1972.

Colman, A., & Colman, L. *Pregnancy: The psychological experience*. New York: The Seabury Press, Inc., 1971.

Fein, R. A. Men's entrance to parenthood. *Family Coordinator*, 1976, *25*, 341–348.

Gilman, R., & Knox, D. Coping with fatherhood: The first year. *Child Psychiatry and Human Development*. 1976, *6*, 134–148.

Gollober, M. A comment on the need for father-infant postpartal interaction. *Journal of Obstetrical, Gynecological and Neonatal Nursing*, 1976, *6*, 17–20.

Greenberg, M., & Morris, N. Engrossment: The newborn's impact upon the father. *American Journal of Orthopsychiatry*, 1974, *44*, 520–531.

Heise, J. Toward better preparation for involved fatherhood. *Journal of Obstetrical, Gynecological and Neonatal Nursing*, 1975, *4*, 32–35.

Hott, J. R. The crisis of expectant fatherhood. *American Journal of Nursing*, 1976, *76*, 1436–1440.

Klaus, M. H., & Kennell, J. H. *Maternal-infant bonding*. Saint Louis: C. V. Mosby Company, 1976.

Kotelchuck, M. *The nature of the child's tie to the father*. Unpublished doctoral dissertation, Harvard University, 1972.

Kotelchuck, M. The infant's relationship to the father: Experimental evidence. In M. E. Lamb (Ed.), *The role of the father in child development*. New York: Wiley, 1976.

Lacoursiere, R. B. Fatherhood and mental illness: A review and new material. *Psychiatric Quarterly*, 1972, *46*, 109–24.

Leonard, S. W. How first-time fathers feel toward their new-borns. *American Journal of Maternal Child Nursing*, 1976, *1*, 361–365.

Lind, R. *Observations after delivery of communications between mother-infant-father*. Paper presented at the International Congress of Pediatrics, Buenos Aires, October, 1974.

McIntire, W. G., Nass, G. D. & Battistone, D. L. Female misperceptions of male parenting attitudes and expectancies. *Youth and Society*, 1974, *6*, 104–111.

Parke, R. D., & O'Leary, S. E. Father/mother/infant interaction in the newborn period: Some findings, some observations, and some unresolved issues. In K. Riegel & J. Meacham (Eds.), *The developing individual in a changing world, Vol. II. Social and environmental issues*. The Hague: Mouton, 1976.

Parke, R. D., O'Leary, S. E., & West, S. *Mother/father/newborn interaction: Effects of maternal medication, labor, and sex of infant.* Proceedings of the American Psychological Association, 1972, 85–86.

Parke, R. D., & Sawin, D. B. The father's role in infancy: A reevaluation. *Family Coordinator,* 1976, *25*, 365–371.

Rendina, I., & Dickerscheid, J. D. Father involvement with first-born infants. *Family Coordinator,* 1976, *25*, 373–378.

Resnick, J. L., Resnick, M. B., Packer, A. B., & Wilson, J. Fathering classes: A psychoeducational model. *The Counseling Psychologist,* 1978, *7*(4), 56–60.

Ritchie, C. A. H., & Swanson, L. A. B. Childbirth outside the hospital—the resurgence of home and clinic deliveries. *American Journal of Maternal Child Nursing,* 1976, *1*, 372–377.

Russell, C. S. Transition to parenthood: Problems and gratification. *Journal of Marriage and the Family,* 1974, *36*, 294–302.

Tanzer, D. *The psychology of pregnancy and childbirth: An investigation of natural childbirth.* Unpublished doctoral dissertation, Brandeis University, 1967.

Trethowan, W. H., & Conlon, M. F. The couvade syndrome. *British Journal of Psychiatry,* 1965, *111*, 57–66.

Fathering Classes:
A Psycho/Educational Model

JAQUELYN L. RESNICK
MICHAEL B. RESNICK
ATHOL B. PACKER
JEN WILSON
University of Florida

Martin's Father (Eichler, 1971) is a children's book that describes a little boy's day with his father, a man actively involved in many aspects of parenting. After being read this story, a six-year-old said "Doesn't Martin have a mother?" We are so accustomed to child care as a woman's domain that we view men who trespass as unusual and try to find reasons for their strange behavior. Responsibility for the care of young children is perhaps the most proscribed sex role in our culture.

The purpose of this paper is to describe the emerging role of fathers in a society that creates conflicts and presents obstacles to men who seek active involvement in fatherhood. A developmental, psycho/educational model will be presented, which enables expectant and new fathers to gain support, knowledge, and skills in their new role and confidence in themselves as fathers.

SOCIALIZATION: A CULTURAL BARRIER TO ACTIVE FATHERING

Taking care of very young children has been pervasively viewed as women's work in the United States. It is reflected in our division of labor on the basis of sex, with women responsible for family and home, and men for the necessary financial support and contact outside the home. Our language is replete with terms that underline the importance of the mother's role: parent surrogates are called "mothering ones"; we study "maternal-infant" bonding; "class mothers" assist in the schools. It is unusual and awkward sounding to hear the words "fathering-one," "paternal-infant" bond, or "class father."

Although motherhood may be losing some of its status, fatherhood has never really been seen as valuable (Kiernan & Scoloveno, 1977). Young boys are rarely encouraged to play at fathering; indeed some are even denied access to dolls. Elementary school textbooks perpetuate the role of fathers as workers outside of the home and uninvolved in the primary care of children (Eaton & Jacobs, 1973). Television often pictures men who do not appear to be serious or competent fathers (Foster, 1964; Hines, 1971). Popular characters like Dagwood Bumstead or Archie Bunker provide children with negative, pathetic, and derisive images of men as fathers.

Professionals in the mental health field have contributed to this restrictive theme. In vocational counseling, women have been asked to choose between a career or a family, or more recently, to consider issues in combining both. In contrast, men are never asked to choose between career and family; rarely are they asked to consider choices that would take into account the demands of combining fatherhood and work. Career counseling has even steered men away from jobs that focus on the care of young children, fields which are overwhelmingly populated by female workers. The message is not a subtle one: man's place is not in the home with children.

Most of the professional literature has focused on mother/child attachments and interactions. The literature which does even mention the father's role frequently also emphasizes some aspect of pathology, such as the negative effects of absentee fathers. A few more recent studies do examine healthy paternal/infant attachment and the impact of the father on child development (Earls, 1976; Greenberg & Morris, 1974; Lamb, 1975, 1976; Lynn, 1975). However, the field is just evolving and requires further research before conclusions can be drawn. New exploration must go beyond simply extending models that have been applied to mother/infant interaction, and focus on fathers as a primary target group.

SEX ROLES AND FATHER IDENTITY

The expected role that father is to play is unclear in the literature. From a physiological perspective, beyond the point of conception, a man is unnecessary. Margaret Mead (1949) went so far as to state that human fatherhood is a social invention. Yet there is some evidence that suggests that men, too, have a desire to nurture, protect, and even give birth to children (Stannard, 1970). The *couvade* is a widespread custom found in disparate primitive societies in which expectant fathers imitate women in labor and even remain in bed once the baby is born, while the new mothers return to work.

The concept of father as more than a biologic necessity is emerging as the psychological aspects of fathering are considered. However, the question remains as to whether or not fathering and mothering functions are different and in what ways.

When male and female roles were more clearly delineated, the father's identity as provider and protector within the family was readily defined, discipline and introducing children to the work outside the home were often his special function. Urbanization has taken the father away from home, with his places of work and recreation often miles away (Hines, 1971). As the father increased time spent away from his family, the paternal model available to the children became increasingly narrowed and intangible (Gollober, 1976). The mother became increasingly powerful, invested with new authority relinquished by the father. In turn, the paternal role has taken on new qualities (love, warmth, compassion). Thus the changes brought about by our advanced technological society have made the affective needs of fathers more important, although we cling to the notion that men function best in the "instrumental" sphere and women in the "expressive" one (Kiernan & Scoloveno, 1977).

An interesting concomitant of father's relative absence from home has been that the young male-child's world is dominated by women, and primary experiences with tenderness, protectiveness, and learning are through relationships with women. Hines (1971) suggests that as the young male identifies with other men, he represses those characteristics he regards as chiefly feminine, a process that cripples or distorts adult responses of fatherliness.

Josselyn (1956) speculated that the division of mothering and fathering functions based on sex-role distinctions are in fact limits due to cultural-economic restrictions. Reiber (1976) speculates that the distinctions are imposed by social norms. Anthropological literature supports the notion that fathers do experience fatherliness as a parallel construct of motherliness and that nurturing characteristics are human characteristics and not for mothers only (Gollober, 1976). In an environment where the feelings of fathers are allowed to be expressed without censure, without fear of embarrassment or accusations of being unmanly, fathers do show evidence of deep warmth, affection, and tenderness for their newborn babies (Hines, 1971).

Social change, especially impetus from the feminist movement has challenged traditional sex-role stereotyped behavior. Androgynous models of mental health (Bem, 1976) have been proposed that support the development of nurturance and sensitivity as characteristics to be valued by men as well as women. Many couples are experimenting with division of labor that is not rigidly sex-role based. More women are entering the work force and to a lesser but noticeable extent, more men are participating in domestic duties including child care. Perhaps the most dramatic change can be seen in the birth process.

EXPECTANT AND NEW FATHERS

In the last decade, there has been an increased number of men (usually middle class) who have chosen to become active participants in the birth of their baby. They attend prenatal classes, where prepared childbirth techniques are taught. The husband and wife function as a team, working through the labor, sharing the birth experience and the often joyous moments afterward. The father can hold and caress his newborn moments after birth, a far cry from the pacer outside in a waiting room being told about the birth by a stranger and seeing his baby through glass windows. In a modification of the Leboyer (1975) method of "gentle birth," the father may bathe his newborn in the delivery room and may even cut the umbilical cord. Although much less common, in a home birth the father may actually assist in or himself deliver the baby.

However, men and women have had to struggle for fathers to be permitted in labor and delivery rooms. In many parts of the country, men are still excluded from labor and delivery rooms by hospital regulations. Once in the labor room, the husband is often viewed as a coach, who should be able to support his wife or not be present. The male is again thrust into the "strong-man" role, not permitted to express anxiety or vulnerability and having to justify his presence at the birth of his child.

Existing versions of family-centered care, with the exception of a handful of birth houses, translate into mother-infant facilities, with fathers granted more or less liberal visiting hours. (This limitation continues as children grow older, with fathers discouraged from overnight visits in pediatric wards.) Despite the advances, when compared with the teaching/learning opportunities available for maternal/infant interaction, father/infant interactions are sadly limited (Gollober, 1976). Whether or not he participates in labor and delivery, the father must deal with his own feelings of impotence in the alien world of the maternity suite, where he may be tolerated or ignored, and feel compelled to control himself during one of life's most overwhelming experiences (Antle, 1975).

In contrast to maternity leave, which is expected and considered necessary, paternity leave is a relatively new concept that has not gained full acceptance. Heise (1975) poignantly describes his attempt to be an involved father, with the ensuing harassment and rejection from friends and relatives who did not comprehend his values. The most traumatic encounter surrounded his paternity leave, which he arranged in spite of accusations that he was taking fatherhood too seriously and insinuations that his wife ought to be able to handle matters by herself. The pain and humiliation he experienced results from a society that better understands personal leave for a death in a family than for a birth, a society that is hostile to the concept of active fathers who feed, bathe, and comfort their children rather than briefly roughhouse with a smiling, powdered little bundle.

TRANSITION TO PARENTHOOD

As a developmental period, expectant and new parenthood has received minimal attention from mental health professionals. The enormity of the change that dramatically disrupts daily life and requires considerable adaptation is matched by the awesome permanence of the change. Short of desertion, a parent is a parent for life. The seemingly unending responsibility for the newborn and its effect on the marital relationships can create unanticipated stress. Many parents are confused by their lack of preparation for parenthood, having underestimated its potential impact.

Although a woman experiences constraints with regard to the mothering role, the pregnancy itself serves as a transitional period during which she is physically and psychologically preparing for childbirth and child rearing. A body of knowledge exists regarding the expectant mother; maturational tasks have been conceptualized and the maternal role is culturally valued. There is no parallel for the expectant father, who not only lacks a clearly defined role, but who must accept pregnancy and subsequent parenthood without concomitant physiological changes to reinforce reality (Antle, 1975).

In fact, some men do experience physical symptoms (the "couvade syndrome") that mimic some aspects of pregnancy (Hott, 1976). There is some question as to whether these symptoms should be viewed as an identification with the pregnant wife or as a result of repressed anxiety and ambivalence regarding the pregnancy. Acknowledgement of any difficulties during the transitional period may be responsible for those men who view such behavior as unmanly.

THE PSYCHO/EDUCATIONAL MODEL

Clearly, our society does not prepare men for active fatherhood, nor does it facilitate the transition. Except for the stereotyped provider/protector role, expressions of early fatherhood are unsupported, the needs of individual men forgotten.

To bridge the gap created by the lack of preparation for fatherhood and the reality of the parental experience, a devolopmental psycho/educational model has been devised (Resnick, Packer, Resnick, & Wilson, 1975). Fathering classes are part of a larger humanistic, interdisciplinary approach to parent/child development education that spans the prenatal period through entry into elementary school. Classes are offered for expectant parents and for parents with infants, toddlers, and preschoolers. The content is both didactic and experiential, based on the evolving needs of developing families.

The classes are led by two members of an interdisciplinary team of counseling psychologists, nurses, child development specialists, and early childhood educators. In the fathering classes, it is advantageous for the leaders to be men and fathers themselves, as they can provide positive and credible role models.

The classes can be taken anytime in the developmental sequence (there are no prerequisites!). Some fathers enter the classes as expectant parents and attend for a year or more, others participate in only one part of the sequence. A few fathers have returned to classes after their second or third child was born. The program has been implemented in a variety of settings (Packer, Resnick, Resnick, & Wilson, 1978; Resnick et al., 1976) offered through university continuing education, the public school system, community mental health agencies, and health care clinics. Class members represent a racial and socioeconomic mix.

EXPECTANT PARENT CLASSES

The expectant parent classes differ from the other classes in that the couple (rather than the father only) participate on a weekly basis. Optimal class size is about six couples or 12 people. Some unmarried couples do attend. It is not uncommon for a few women to attend without their spouse; rarely do men attend alone.

Information about labor and delivery and instruction in prepared childbirth techniques are focal points of the class (and most likely represent the identified need that attracts class members). The men seem to be most comfortable seeking information and learning useful tasks they can perform during labor and delivery. They are willing to ask questions that are externally focused, such as "what can my wife do about leg cramps?" but tend to be more reticent when the focus is on their own feelings and needs.

It is helpful to occasionally break up the class into same-sex groups. The men seem to have an easier time dealing with issues surrounding roles, expectations, and competency (or lack of it) when not in the presence of women. One man's disclosure on a previously taboo subject can create an atmosphere for mutual sharing. For example, one expectant father talked about his wife's plans to breast feed in public and his disgusted, angry reaction. His candor enabled others to examine their feelings regarding breast feeding and their relative comfort/discomfort with the issues involved.

The group sharing provides the expectant father with a forum to express concerns and ask for help. It also introduces some issues of which he might not have been aware prior to this time. Reality testing occurs as he identifies his opinions and checks them out with other group members, who may have a very different perspective. Support is offered for the wide range of options available. An appreciation develops for the numerous ways in which fatherhood can be enacted.

Typical concerns brought out by expectant fathers in class include: fears that their wife might die or that their baby will be somehow deformed; fears of inadequacy or dependency complicated by the need to deny such feelings and appear strong; feeling rejected or neglected by their wife; having to adjust to new modes and/or decreased frequency of sexual expression. Some men feel threatened or trapped by a sense that pleasures are being exchanged for responsibilities at a rapid pace.

The class stresses the importance of developing decision-making skills, since many critical decisions must be made at this time. Open communication within the couple is practiced and assertive training is introduced, if appropriate. These skills are particularly important as the couple determines for themselves their identity as parents as they interface with hospital staff, friends, relatives, and employers and as they relate to each other. Role playing that anticipates difficult situations assists the couple in developing effective methods of handling targeted problems.

Class members are taken on a tour of the maternity suite to acquaint them with the procedures they will go through and familiarize them with the surroundings, diffusing fears of the unknown. Another aspect of the reality testing involves visits to the class by new parents, selected for their willingness to share their experiences and concerns openly. The expectant parents are also invited to attend a session of the parent/infant classes. These interactions with real parents and infants—perhaps the most exciting part of the class—provide concrete models of the transition process.

FATHERING CLASSES

Classes for fathers meet for two hours on a monthly or biweekly basis, on a weeknight or Saturday morning. Perhaps the most unique aspect of the class is that the fathers attend together with their infants. Classes are groups according to the child's age (under 6 months, 6–12 months, 12–24 months, or preschool age). The optimal class size is about eight fathers (16 fathers and babies).

The first part of the class is devoted to knowledge and skills concerning infant development. Fathers and infants participate in structured physical development exercises together and with other class members. These learning activities have several purposes:

1. To establish basic communication patterns between fathers and infants;
2. To facilitate infant's sensory-motor, cognitive, and affective development;
3. To teach fathers to take cues from their infants and become aware of their unique and everchanging behavioral repertoires;
4. To provide fathers with opportunities to handle infants and develop primary care skills;
5. To encourage the use of natural caretaking situations such as feeding, bathing, diapering,and so forth, as opportunities for positive interaction that will enhance father/child relationships and infant's growth and development. (For more information regarding the exercises, see Resnick, Packer, Resnick, & Wilson, 1976.)

The second part of the class is the sharing period, where the men have an opportunity to focus on themselves. The process resembles a small group organized around homogeneous concerns—in this case, the impact of fatherhood. The men discuss both positive and negative feelings about their new role and how it has affected their everyday lives. Their relationships with their wives, concerns about sexuality, relationships with parents, inlaws or other family members, relationships with their other children, fatigue, anxiety, and jealously are typical topics. The content of this part of class is determined entirely by the needs of the members.

Some men feel pressured by the demands of work, followed by unexpected demands at home to help with the baby, assist with housework, or attend to emotional needs of their spouse. Unanticipated expenses related to the newborn can create financial woes, exacerbated if their wife had contributed to the income and stopped. If both parents work, other difficulties may arise concerning child care, time management and exhaustion.

New fathers often describe their frustration in finding enough time alone with their wives. They may feel displaced by the new baby and resentful of its ever-present intrusions. Some men are insensitive to their wife's conflicting roles; others understand the situation too well and feel guilty about their own feelings. The men often request help in communication skills, particularly in terms of effective fighting. Many men also find it difficult to spend enough time with their babies (the average father spends less than 10 minutes per day with his child). Attending class with their baby often represents the most time the two spend together.

Although beyond the scope of this paper, special issues involving divorced fathers, step-fathers, unmarried fathers, and widowed fathers must also be considered. These men are welcome in the classes and have been readily integrated. However, classes specifically aimed at these groups would also be appropriate.

Particular problems can be presented and the group along with the leaders work together to resolve the issues. Sometimes the focus of the problem is infant oriented—for example, what to do with an irritable baby. Other times there is a personal focus, such as handling of feelings of sexual rejection. As in other groups, the shared concerns, the knowledge that others are vulnerable, and the support offered serves to encourage these men as they seek to develop their identities as fathers. Response repertoires are increased with regard to specific parenting situations. The father is seen as part of a triadic (or larger) family interaction, with complex needs and communication patterns to be considered. Particular styles or theories of parenting are not embraced. Rather, the men are taught to develop confidence in themselves as fathers and to feel valued and important in that role.

In addition to class, fathers can participate in a toy-lending library and occasional toy-making workshops. The class also serves as a first level of identification of parents or children who need more specialized help. Referrals are made to community agencies when health or psychosocial problems are observed that require supplemental services.

IMPLICATIONS

Expectant and new fatherhood are anticipated life events that may be particularly stressful for men because of their lack of preparation and clearly defined role expectations, their lack of exposure to specific information regarding this period, and the great personal change they must undergo with little institutional or societal support.

The purpose of the fathering program described is to involve fathers early in their new role, at a time that may be critical for developing attachments with their newborn (Klaus & Kennel, 1976; Greenberg & Morris, 1974). A combination of emotional support and specific information is essential since both aspects are currently unavailable to a majority of men. Feedback from a wide range of fathers indicates their relief and appreciation for a program that attends to their very real needs, that allows them exposure to other fathers and young children, and removes them from their isolation in fatherhood.

Combining work and fatherhood becomes a serious issue, requiring basic social change to make active fathering viable. The male trap (Clinebell, 1977) of achievement through the all-consuming work ethic is incompatible with active involvement in fathering, although our present system externally rewards such success. The fathers in class have been surprised to discover parts of themselves that had never been expressed; paternal feelings of love, tenderness, and joy in their interactions with their children. A bond developed that is much more intimate than one resulting from the provider/protector role and that is intrinsically rewarding to them.

Psycho/educational programs are needed to facilitate men's transition to fatherhood as a preventive and proactive model. Without intervention during this developmental period, men will continue to be locked into their stereotypic roles, possibly remote or alienated from their children. Other consequences more alarming to society in general are the reported increases in family dissolution, male sexually deviant behavior (Hott, 1976), and child abuse during this stressful time. When prepared and educated about the possibilities, men respond enthusiastically to the invitation to become involved fathers. The problem to date has been that few have been extended a serious invitation.

REFERENCES

Antle, K. Psychologic involvement in pregnancy by expectant fathers. *JOGN Nursing*, 1975, *4*, 40–42.

Bem, S. Beyond androgyny: Some presumptuous prescriptions for a liberated sexual identity. In A. V. Kaplan & J. P. Bean (Eds.), *Beyond sex-role stereotypes: Readings toward a psychology of androgyny*. Boston: Little, Brown, 1976.

Clinebell, H. Creative fathering: The problems and potentialities of changing sex roles. In E. V. Stein (Ed.), *Fathering: Fact or fable*. Nashville: Abingdon, 1977.

Earls, F. The fathers (not the mothers): Their importance and influence with infants and young children. *Psychiatry,* 1976, *39,* 209–227.

Eaton, C., & Jacobs, C. Changing the textbooks. *American Education,* 1973, *9,* 26–28.

Eichler, M. *Martin's father.* Chapel Hill, N.C.: Lollipop Power, 1971.

Foster, J. E. Father in ages: Television and the idea. *Journal of Marriage and the Family,* 1964, *26,* 353–356.

Gollober, M. A comment on the need for father/infant postpartal interaction. *JOGN Nursing,* 1976, *5,* 17–20.

Greenberg, M., & Morris, N. Engrossment: The newborn's impact upon the father. *American Journal of Orthopsychiatry,* 1974, *44,* 520–531.

Heise, J. Toward better preparation for involved fatherhood. *JOGN Nursing,* 1975, *4,* 32–35.

Hines, J. D. Father—the forgotten man. *Nursing Forum,* 10, 1971, 177–200.

Hott, J. R. The crisis of expectant fatherhood. *American Journal of Nursing,* 1976, *76,* 1436–1440.

Josselyn, I. M. Cultural forces, motherliness, and fatherliness. *American Journal of Orthopsychiatry,* 1956, *26,* 264–271.

Kiernan, B., & Scoloveno, M. A. Fathering. *Nursing Clinics of North America,* 1977, *12,* 481–490.

Klaus, M., & Kennell, J. *Maternal-infant bonding.* New York: Mosby Press, 1976.

Lamb, M. E. Fathers: Forgotten contributors to child development. *Human Development,* 1975, *18,* 245–266.

Lamb, M. E. *The role of the father in child development.* New York: Wiley, 1976.

Leboyer, F. *Birth without violence.* New York: Knopf, 1975.

Lynn, D. *The father: His role in child development.* Monterey, Calif: Brooks/Cole, 1975.

Mead, M. *Male and female.* New York: Dell, 1949.

Packer, A. B., Resnick, M. B., Resnick, J. L., & Wilson, J. An elementary school with parents and infants: A model parenting education program. *Young Children,* 1978, in press.

Reiber, V. D. Is the nurturing role natural to fathers? *Maternal/Child Nursing.* 1976, *1,* 366–371.

Resnick, M. B., Packer, A. B., Resnick, J. L., & Wilson, J. *Alachua County Parenting Education Program.* Final Report to the Office of Education, Department of Health, Education, and Welfare. Grant No. 007503-188, 1976.

Resnick, M. B., Packer, A. B., Wilson, J., & Resnick, J. L. Parenting education: An interdisciplinary model. *Dimensions: Journal of the Southern Association of Children Under Six,* 1975, *3,* 4–9.

Stannard, V. Adam's rib, or the woman within. *Trans-Action,* 1970, *8,* 52–59.

Fathers with
Child Custody

ROBERT H. WOODY
University of Nebraska at Omaha

State child-custody statutes are increasingly being directed toward the concept of the best interests of the child (as opposed to the best interests of all persons concerned). Impetus for this trend came, in part, from a manifesto presented by the Uniform State Child Custody Jurisdiction Act (Commissioners on Uniform State Laws, 1969). This Act was adopted by the American Bar Association in the fall of 1968, but it remains, of course, for each state to implement it through legislation (an elaboration of the Act has been provided by Bodenheimer, 1969). In brief, the American Bar Association's Family Law Section (1973) interprets that Act as supporting that the welfare of children is primary and that the terms of legal separation or dissolution of a marriage relevant to child support, custody, and visitation must satisfy the court as "being fair and reasonable" and as promoting "the best interests of the child" (p. 151). A social and psychological rationale for the best interests of the child concept has been posited by Goldstein, Freud, and Solnit (1973); this rationale strongly emphasizes the important differences between the "biological" parent and the "psychological" parent, asserts the biological parent has less influence than the psychological parent, and proposes than the best interests of the child potentially extend beyond an allegiance to biological parents.

As might be anticipated, the shift to the best interests of the child concept has led to questioning of the existing child-custody practices. It has been estimated that at least 60% of all divorces affect young children (Westman, Cline, & Kramer, 1970), and there is reason to believe that the percentage is increasing. Of interest, it appears that fewer than 2% of contested divorces were over the custody of children, but to date there are no data available on the actual number of child-custody decisions contested.

Over the past century, the trend in American child-custody decisions has been clearly to give priority to the mother. Slovenko (1973) states:

> The father as a rule recognizes that the mother can render better care, the children usually wish to be with the mother, and consequently he does not request child custody or possession of the family home in the

divorce action. The mother is literally the housekeeper. It is observable among human and animal species that it is generally the mother who cares for and protects the young. The father may also recognize that a custody dispute is a futile endeavor. Surveys of sample cases indicate that maternal custody is awarded to 85 to 95% of the cases [p. 361].

Ploscowe, Foster, and Freed (1972) also indicate that the mother gets custody in the majority of the instances; they estimate that the mother receives custody in approximately 80% of the cases, the father in 10% of the cases, and both parents (joint custody) or relatives are made guardians for the other 10% of the children.

DISCRIMINATION AGAINST FATHERS

The heavy reliance upon mothers for custody creates the question of possible sexism; that is, there is the question of whether preference is given to a parent in child-custody proceedings because of the parent's sex, not because of the issues directly relevant to custody. As cited elsewhere (Woody, 1977 b), research on a sample of lawyers, psychiatrists, psychologists, and social workers supported that professionals do not *generally* apply significant differences to the criteria that they believe are important for evaluating a mother for suitability for custody as opposed to evaluating the father for suitability for custody. In other words, there did not seem to be a consistent ''doublestandard'' in the degree of importance attributed to a particular factor according to the sex of the parent. There were, however, a variety of subtle distinctions made, and many of these seemed to be attributed to the professional's discipline, age, marital history, and related demographic factors. The data seemed to support that the sex of the parent alone does not generally preordain the professional's views about the placement decision. The implications are that mothers and fathers will be evaluated without obvious sex bias and, consequently, that fathers may be receiving custody in a greater number of cases than in the past.

PREFERENCE FOR FATHERS

Historically, there was a time when fathers received priority in child-custody determinations. Under early common law, the father was deemed to have the primary right to children, including ''children of tender years'' (in more recent times, the criterion of ''tender years'' was the basis for awarding children to the mother). For example, in the 1800s, children were viewed as property and the male was the only one entitled to possess property; therefore, children were automatically seen as being under the aegis of the father. Given the agricultural nature of society, children had monetary value and their status as chattel provided the father with additional wealth.

Even in those early days the courts were prone to make sure that the child's welfare was cared for. Just before the turn of the 20th century, common-law practice led to a shift toward the mother receiving custody of children, particularly those of "tender years," as long as she had not been shown "to be morally unfit or otherwise unsuitable," and this practice was based, supposedly, on the best interests of the child. Court decisions strongly reflect moral considerations; the usual form of these is that unless the mother is proven to be morally unfit, she is "entitled to preference as the legal guardian." As a clear illustration of special preference for the mother over the father, an eight-year-old boy had been in the custody of his father for four years when his mother petitioned for custody; both parents were considered fit for custody, but the lower courts held for the mother "to the effect that children should have as much of the companionship with their mother as possible because there is no satisfactory substitute for her care and nothing so helpful as her love." The Supreme Court, however, reversed for the father, citing the facts that a close relationship existed between the boy and the father, that they engaged in numerous activities ("These shared activities promote Tommy's welfare and development by providing him with the companionship necessary if he is to give him expression to his youthful energies"), and that the paternal grandmother (who resided with her son and grandson) compensated "with a good deal of love and affection." In conclusion, the Supreme Court stated: "He can enjoy his mother's love and attention only at the expense of substantial loss of his father's companionship"—and this loss was deemed to be too heavy a price to pay (Fish versus Fish, 1968).

Traditionally, the courts have applied the "fitness test" in child custody decisions—that is, one parent is, in effect, declared "unfit." Obviously negative psychological consequences can result when one parent is branded unfit, and this label could adversely affect the child's subsequent relationship with that parent. With enlightenment, recent court actions are supporting a "better fit" concept. There is no attempt to establish "unfitness." Thus, even when both parents exhibit genuine love and affection for the children, have not been neglectful of their parental duties, and are generally fit for continued meeting of the children's needs, the court decision focuses on which parent is most able to meet the best interests of the child. From the onset, this judicial conceptualization has offered new opportunity for fathers to receive custody (Solomon, 1977).

DEVELOPMENTAL IMPLICATIONS

From the viewpoint of developmental psychology, it is clear that the unique relationship of the child with each parent influences the child's psychosocial development. Krech and Crutchfield (1948) cite extensive research evidence linking the development of social beliefs and attitudes to a person's family life. There seems no doubt that the disruption caused by the stress of divorce and the possible deleterious effects of being placed with only one parent, be it the father or the mother, could readily influence the social development of the child in the area of beliefs, attitudes, group roles, and more broadly, social behavior.

Of importance to counseling theory, the impact on a child's self-esteem caused by divorce and the ensuing absence of one parent is noteworthy. Kleinfeld (1970) states that the "psychological and sociological literature on divorce seems fairly united behind the proposition that divorce tends to reduce children's self-esteem in inverse proportion to the children's ages" (p. 239); he further elaborates on this position: "Some of the relations between the effect on self-esteem and the age of the children has been explained as meaning that a child during the Oedipal period more than other developmental stages interprets the divorce as punishment for his hostility toward his parents or as a fulfillment of fantasy wishes that are more pronounced at that time, and so he feels guilty" (p. 329).

Related to self-esteem is the need for nurturance, and the removal of either parent through custody determinations can jeopardize the sources of nurturing for the child. Although the mother has traditionally fulfilled the primary nurturant role, as reflected by Lidz's (1968) argument that "the mother is the primary and major nurturant figure to the child, particularly the small child" (p. 56), the unquestioned linkage of self-esteem to identification would support that children of either sex could be adversely influenced by the deprivation of contact—for example, opportunity for identification, with either parent. Thus, the tradition of placing the child with the mother stood to deprive the child of an opportunity for identification with the father.

Heretofore, the custody decisions have generally produced situations in which mothers received custody and fathers tended to become absent from the family system. Consequently, research has focused on the father's absence and primarily on its effects on boys. Mussen, Conger, and Kagan (1969) assert: "Perhaps not surprisingly—in view of the importance of the same-sex parent as an identification model—absence of the same-sex parent appears particularly important" (p. 493). In other words, the tradition of preferring mothers for custody places boys in a particularly vulnerable position regarding masculine identification. Mussen, Conger, and Kagan (1969) further recognize the importance of the age of the separation of the boy from the father, and suggest "that boys who lose their father early, before identification can be assumed to have been clearly established, have greater difficulty in establishing a masculine sex-role identification and acquiring sex-type traits, whereas absence of the father after the child reaches age five has far less effect" (p. 494).

As might be anticipated, research on parental absence (including the absence of only one parent) reveals that there are more broken homes in the backgrounds of delinquents and children suffering from emotional disorders than in nondisturbed children and that school performance often suffers in children subjected to divorce and/or separation of their parents (Mussen, Conger, & Kagan, 1969). Likewise, it is well documented that parental absence, which could lead to affect deprivation, can lead to psychotoxic and emotional deficiency diseases (Watson, 1959). Kleinfeld (1970) asserts that the divorce of their parents often leads children to decreased self-esteem and to behavior problems. Although definitive research is lacking, evidence is mounting that the divorce process has a deleterious effect on the emotional and behavioral adjustment of both children and adults, and that professionals have yet to recognize the need to provide services unique to problems stemming from divorce.

COUNSELING INTERVENTIONS

The essence of the "best interests of the child concept" prescribes that various factors be evaluated to ascertain which parent is the better able to meet the needs of the child. These factors reflect educational, psychological, social, medical, and cultural dimensions. This concept clearly creates a mandate for greater behavioral science involvement in the evaluation, notably as would be provided through the services of professional psychologists (Woody, 1977b).

To date the role of the counseling psychologist in child custody cases is ill defined. The following are ten recommendations designed to establish an operational set for the counseling psychologist that will assure a high level of professional conduct, incorporate necessary legal considerations, and accommodate a healthful advocacy for all parties concerned.

First, *the counseling psychologist should be open to parenting alternatives.* It is naive to assume that the counseling psychologist or any other professional is free from biased notions about parenting. The law is clear: the best interests of the child are paramount and neither parent has an automatic right to custody. The tradition of placement with the mother is subject to question, but all professionals have experienced the societal conditioning that produces the view that mothers have an inalienable right to custody. Although legally this view is indefensible, even judges are not immune to it; for example, one judge recently stated, in effect: "I know what the law says, but as long as I am judge, children will be placed with their mother, because a mother can care for a child a lot better than a father!" Similarly, research on lawyers, psychiatrists, psychologists, and social workers reveals clear-cut tendencies to maintain different criteria when dealing with a mother versus a father (Woody, 1977a, 1977c). Counseling psychologists must guard against permitting their personal values to dictate parenting options.

Second, *the counseling psychologist should be able to help the most able parent, which could easily be the father, vigorously pursue a legal decision.* Solomon (1977), in the context of "the fathers' revolution in custody cases," points out the father's need for professional help in counteracting bias on the part of the judge: "Since we have not yet reached that stage in custody litigation in which judges are willing to veer away from their traditional bias toward mothers, a father and his lawyer must have the courage to challenge a judge's objectivity at the trial" (p. 36). Certainly this principle extends to the father's counseling psychologist, who might be providing expert testimony in the legal proceedings vis-a-vis the father's capabilities for meeting needs unique to the particular child. Elsewhere (Woody, 1978), a detailed strategy has been set forth to help parents effectively integrate consultants, such as counseling psychologists, into the case.

Third, and related to the first recommendation, *the counseling psychologist should be prepared to maintain an objective stance.* Involvement must be removed from personal ego needs. Any personal experience that could impact upon professional functioning in child-custody cases, such as a divorce or custody dispute within the counseling psychologist's personal life, must be worked through prior to providing child-custody services.

Fourth, *the counseling psychologist should offer evaluative information from a scientific base.* Assessment methods must be reasonably objective. The criteria underlying judgments about parenting potential must have a solid rationale and be specified beforehand. Safeguards must be maintained to assure adequate reliability and validity for the evaluation. The systems for interpreting and communicating the data must be well defined.

Fifth, *the counseling psychologist should be a family advocate.* In this age of concern for children's rights, it is easy to be caught up in the fervor of atoning for past denigration of children. Also, being employed by one of the parents sets the stage for the counseling psychologist to act on behalf of the parent. Even if the father (or mother) is clearly the best able to meet the needs of the child, the advocacy should not be for the parent or child per se. The long-range goal is an overall family life that will be in the best interests of the child and that will be healthful and life-enhancing for all persons therein. Thus, professional advocacy should emphasize the conditions—present and future—that will contribute to achieving this goal. The focus on health, as opposed to pathology, has long been a distinguishing feature of counseling psychology, and there is, therefore, a natural link between family advocacy and the specialty of counseling psychology.

Sixth, *the counseling psychologist should help the father prepare for and adapt to the new parenting relationship with his child.* Because of the sexist role reinforcers to which all Americans are subjected, it is probable that every father will have preconceived notions about what parenting does and does not entail. Bernstein (1977) has provided a helpful list of areas with which the lawyer and counselor can assist the father in preparation for child custody. It is necessary to help the father come to grips with the requirements of day-to-day living (for example, day care, laundry, and so forth), as well as with gaining awareness of his own and the child's emotional and behavioral needs. In a study of fathering after marital separation, Keshet and Rosenthal (1978) reveal a host of logistical and psychological problems typically encountered in single fathering. Essentially, the counseling psychologist should strive to help the father: (1) acquire a totally new framework for competently fulfilling parenting responsibilities; and (2) use the single fathering experience as an opportunity for growth for both himself and his children.

Seventh, *the counseling psychologist should give special attention to facilitating a more comprehensive father/child relationship, especially relevant to communication.* Both the father and child will be under pressure to fulfill needs in their newly defined relationship, without the wife/mother in the household, and this is likely to sorely test the relationship. As has been established throughout human relations, communication channels must be open and efficient. The nature of counseling lends support to achieving these relationship goals.

Eighth, *the counseling psychologist should encourage proper future contacts, as might be in the best interests of the child, between the father and mother.* The divorce and the winning/losing of child custody does not end any relationships. Rather, it is a redefining of the relationships. Consequently, it is inevitable that all persons in the family will experience conflicts about their new relationships. Although counseling cannot always be asserted to both the mother and father (that is, postdivorce counseling), there are many divorced couples who welcome a counselor's helping them adjust to their unmarried state. Regardless, in keeping with family advocacy, the mother and father should be encouraged to work together to plan the boundaries and guidelines for their future sharing of parental responsibility for the child. To lose custody does not abrogate parental responsibility; it delimits the responsibility of each parent, but the child's welfare often depends upon continuing contact with both parents. Counseling can help the parents: (1) to recognize their shared commitment; (2) to gain control over neurotic impulses (for example, to get revenge on each other at the expense of the children), (3) to learn from their past marriage (thereby promoting better future relationships, such as in remarriage), and (4) to arrange for ongoing fulfillment of the best interests of the child.

Nine, *the counseling psychologist should assure that institutional restrictions do not jeopardize professional services to the family.* There are schools, agencies, hospitals, universities, and so on that assign certain functions to the counseling psychologist but preclude others that are integrally related. For example, one counseling psychologist described how he was required to evaluate children, including those for child-custody cases, but was prohibited by the hospital's policies from counseling with the parents about the findings (he was only allowed to briefly interpret the test data to the parents and to submit a written report to a referring physician).

This restricted role definition might be acceptable, assuming that other professionals are available and able to provide parent counseling. In this instance, such was not the case; there was virtually no parent counseling or follow-up service. This arrangement could easily prove to be a disservice, namely by leaving persons without guidance after they had been subject to psychological provocation. Indeed, this could be viewed as unethical behavior. The counseling psychologist should preface involvement in child-custody legal proceedings with administrative arrangements that will assure that a comprehensive professional service is available to the parents and child. This may mean the creation of a new job definition.

Tenth, *the counseling psychologist must gain adequate professional training in child custody.* Few, if any, counseling psychology training programs routinely include in-depth exposure to the socio-legal factors that have relevance to a counseling psychologist's working in child custody. A basic academic knowledge of the American legal system, with special references to domestic law (for example, state statutes and common-law cases for divorce and child custody), is required. Theories of marriage, divorce, and parenting should be covered. Self-understanding of how the counseling psychologist's personal characteristics could influence percepts and actions is mandatory for all types of counseling problems, and in child custody it is especially crucial. Assessment methods must be objective and directly connected to child custody considerations. On-going training opportunities, to keep the counselor knowledgeable about current trends in legal decisions and alternatives for remedies, are essential.

SUMMARY

The best interests of the child concept and laws prescribing equal rights for both parents usher in an era where more fathers will be receiving custody of their children. They will need professional help to adapt to their new parenting roles. With its focus on health, counseling psychology must assume a prominent place in child-custody legal proceedings. To properly work with fathers in child-custody cases, the counseling psychologist should:

1. Be open to parenting alternatives;
2. Be able to help the most able parent, which could easily be the father, vigorously pursue a legal decision;
3. Be prepared to maintain an objective stance;
4. Offer evaluative information from a scientific base;
5. Be a family advocate (not an advocate for the child or a parent);
6. Help the father prepare for and adapt to the new parenting responsibilities;
7. Give special attention to facilitating a more comprehensive father/child relationship, especially relevant to communication;

8. Encourage proper future contacts, as might be in the best interest of the child, between the father and mother;
9. Assure that institutional restrictions do not jeopardize professional services to the family; and
10. Gain adequate professional training in child custody.

The decision to seek and accept child custody, be it by the mother or father, is a critical one. Our society has established support sources (financial, psychological, social) for mothers with custody, but to date the rarity of fathers receiving custody has left a void in support sources for them. The need exists, however, and is likely to increase, for comprehensive counseling services being available to fathers facing child-custody legal proceedings. Professional responsibility issues a challenge for counseling psychologists to step forward with services for these fathers.

REFERENCES

American Bar Association Family Law Section. Proposed Revised Uniform Marriage and Divorce Act. *Family Law Quarterly,* 1973, *7*, 135–167.

Bernstein, B. E. Lawyer and counselor as an interdisciplinary team: Preparing the father for custody. *Journal of Marriage and Family Counseling,* 1977, *3*(3), 29–40.

Bodenheimer, B. M. The Uniform Child Custody Jurisdiction Act. *Family Law Quarterly,* 1969, *3*, 304–316.

Commissioners on Uniform State Laws. Uniform Child Custody Jurisdiction Act. *Family Law Quarterly,* 1969, *3*, 317–330.

Fish versus Fish (Supreme Court of Minnesota, 1968), 280 Minn. 316, 159NW2d 71.

Goldstein, J., Freud, A., & Solnit, A. J. *Beyond the best interest of the child.* New York: Free Press, 1973.

Keshet, H. F., & Rosenthal, K. M. Fathering after marital separation. *Social Work,* 1978, *23*, 11–18.

Kleinfeld, A. J. The balance of power among infants, their parents, and the state. *Family Law Quarterly,* 1970, *4*, 320–350.

Krech, D., & Crutchfield, R. S. *Theory and problems of social psychology.* New York: McGraw-Hill, 1948.

Lidz, T. *The person: His development throughout the life cycle.* New York: Basic Books, 1968.

Mussen, P. H., Conger, J. J., & Kagan, J. *Child development and personality* (3rd ed.). New York: Harper & Row, 1969.

Ploscowe, M., Foster, H. H., Jr., & Freed, D. J. *Family law: Cases and materials* (2nd ed.). Boston: Little, Brown, 1972.

Slovenko, R. *Psychiatry and law.* Boston: Little, Brown, 1973.

Solomon, P. F. Parents' rights: The fathers' revolution in custody cases. *Trial,* 1977, *13*(10), 33–37.

Watson, R. I. *Psychology of the child: Personal, social, and disturbed child development.* New York: Wiley, 1959.

Westman, J. C., Cline, D. W., & Kramer, D. A. Role of child psychiatry in divorce. *Archives of General Psychiatry,* 1970, *23*, 416–420.

Woody, R. H. Behavioral sciences criteria in child-custody determinations. *Journal of Marriage and Family Counseling,* 1977, *3*, 11–18. (a)

Woody, R. H. Psychologists in child custody. In D. D. Sales (Ed.), *Psychology in the legal process.* New York: Spectrum, 1977, 249–267. (b)

Woody, R. H. Sexism in child custody decisions. *Personnel and Guidance Journal,* 1977, *56,* 168–170. (c)

Woody, R. H. *Getting custody: Winning the last battle of the marital war.* New York: Macmillan, 1978

Communication Strategies for Males Following the Death of a Child

JOHN WANZENRIED
University of Nebraska

It is now recognized that the conspiracy of silence about death and dying has been vanquished. Within the last few years, death—with its effect on the living and dying—has been the subject for discussion and research. Recent accounts deal with the process of dying, the process of grief, the effects of death on the living (for example, Kübler-Ross, 1969; Bergman, 1974).

This paper examines the grief process of the male parent suffering the death of a child. The intervention strategies that are here explained have evolved from the author's extensive experience with counselors and parents of Sudden-Infant-Death-Syndrome (SIDS) children.

Sudden Infant Death Syndrome, the leading cause of death in infants after the first week of life, is the sudden, unexplained death of a healthy infant. The effect of this unpredictable and unpreventable disease on parents, as well as on friends and relatives, can be emotionally devastating. It is an event that can never be fully comprehended by those who have experienced it, much less by those who serve as their counselors. And, the availability of research specifically dealing with the unique problems of parents who grieve from Sudden Infant Death loss is minimal. The unique nature of the *untimely death of a child* makes research difficult and, for this same reason, makes research imperative.

Systematic longitudinal studies, such as those conducted on terminally ill cancer patient families, cannot be replicated with Sudden-Infant-Death parents. All of the communication surrounding the death of the child begins with the totally unpredicted death of the child. Death from old age or terminal illness allows resolution-focused communication to take place gradually. This period of preparation for death is not, of course, available to parents who suffer the precipitous loss of a child. Furthermore, attention in the form of counseling cannot begin until the crisis of unexpected death occurs.

LANGUAGE AND SELF-DEFINITION

A person is inextricably bound up in the words used for self-definition. Changes in self-perception are a naturally occurring, voluntary process. The exception to the slow voluntary change occurs in crisis situations. When a crisis occurs, an individual does not have the option of deciding whether or not he/she will change; change is inevitable. The crisis that occurs in the external environment generates a concomitant internal change in self-definition.

For the parent who loses a child, the words used for self-definition change immediately. No longer is he/she simply a parent; he/she is now a parent of a dead baby. Changes in the individual's self-perception and changes in the perceptions others have of that self occur instantaneously. The precipitous nature of the change engendered by the event of SIDS, or other accidental death, necessitates awareness by the professional and volunteer personnel who work with people in crises.

Language stereotyping can create unrealistic generalizations against which individuals measure themselves and against which the individual is measured by significant others. Bergman (1974) related:

> a Seattle pediatrician lost her baby to Sudden Infant Death Syndrome in the past year and had an unusually severe grief/guilt reaction. This was alleviated only after she was treated as a grieving mother rather than as a fellow pediatrician [p. 119].

The example vividly demonstrates the power of language labels (that is, to be a "mother," not a "doctor") and their influence on behavior and attitude. The cultural language definitions, which prescribe human behavior during grief, can have devastating consequences for those males who are unable to conform to those definitions. A father's perceived need to present a socially approved image, such as a stereotyped "macho" facade (in which no emotional disruptions are permissible), can create dissonance between what is emotionally experienced and the expected behavior defined by language stereotyping.

Much of the difficulty males experience in coping with the grief after the loss of a child stems from the necessity of maintaining a facade of strength. From a cultural standpoint, males are not typically allowed the freedom to express emotions as freely as women. The internalization of this normative standard forces men to grieve in solitude. Such isolation creates a number of difficulties, one of which is the lack of verbalization of feelings and sharing of those feelings with others. Emotional venting allows access to and understanding of feelings. In tandem with sensitive counseling, affective verbal sharing serves as a cathartic release of emotional tensions conducive to positive mental health.

Parents, regardless of sex, differ in their reactions to the sudden death of a child, and herein lies the basis for an important conceptualization regarding etiology of emotional disruption; that is, the parental reaction to childhood death can best be characterized as a "traumatic neurosis," and counseling interventions should be tailored accordingly. Fenichel (1945) states, "All neurotic phenomena are based on insufficiencies of the normal control apparatus" (p. 19); and, thus, parents with extreme reactions to a child's death can be assumed to be lacking in reserve ego strength adequate for the task of coping with the loss of their child. In other words, "too much excitation enters the mental apparatus in a given unit of time and cannot be mastered; such experiences are called traumatic" (Fenichel, 1945, p. 19).

In the case of childhood death, each parent has a given amount of ego strength (which depends on the person's overall life patterns, such as personality development and the effectiveness of ego defense mechanisms). The events associated with the child's death send forth stimuli that produce excitation in the organism. The duration and intensity of the excitation determines whether the reserve ego strength is adequate or inadequate; and when it is inadequate, there is extreme emotional flooding and a transitory deterioration of ego functioning.

COUNSELING STRATEGY

Following the traumatic neurosis model, counseling interventions should have three emphases (Fenichel, 1945; Woody, 1978). First, *getting distance* allows the parents to rest and avoid more stress in order to collect energy; distancing from locations and events associated with the death helps the person reactivate ego functions, such as intellect and logic, to the pretrauma state and provides an opportunity to re-establish psychological equilibrium. This is called the "quieting down" method. Second, *belated discharge* of actions or emotions can be beneficial (but painful), and professional guidance is essential to "let it all out." This is the "stormy" method. Third, *catharsis*, a method rooted in communications, can be constructive. The risk of secondary gains during the ventilation of feelings must be avoided. The counseling psychologist may allow a degree of passivity and dependency and give honest reassurance and "take it easy" suggestions, yet constantly structure the interactions to progressively lead the parent back toward self-responsibility and management of emotions and behavior.

Difficulties may arise from the father's withholding of grief. The mother, observing no visible signs of grief, may infer that her husband is not experiencing the intense grief she knows. This situation poses the "Catch 22" problem for the father. Fearing that his expression of devastation over the lost child will create more pain for his wife, who may feel her entire world is crumbling, the husband withholds. Observing this reserve, the wife questions the intensity and genuineness of her husband's grief.

The counselor's strategy should be to help the father understand, via introspection and clarification, his wife's perceptions of his actions. The counselor must demonstrate how the withholding of emotions creates difficulties for both the father and the mother—for the mother, in that her perceptions of the reasons for her spouse's behavior are inaccurate, and for the father, in that he feels forced to divorce his feelings from his actions. From involvement with many cases, it seems that when the husband related his painful feelings, his wife is astounded and remarks that she never realized her husband was experiencing them. In fact, it is not uncommon for the wife to accidentally discover her husband grieving "in the basement" or "in the garage"—some place where he can exhibit grief without upsetting her. Although women may react to the death with overt crying, men often vent grief through anger. This anger can be projected at things, at people, or at events. It is only through the mutual understanding and sharing of the grief that resolution may take place. Thus, a couple counseling format is desirable.

Traditionally, the burden for childrearing falls to the mother: thus, the responsibility for the infant's well-being lies with her. Because of the unusual nature of the Sudden Infant Death Syndrome, for example, the advent of the disease often leaves many unanswered questions, not the least of which is: Was the parent responsible, negligent, careless? Similar questions arise in the event of accidental death. Authorities may say that there was no evidence of negligence or irresponsibility, but if the baby's death is not accepted as a nonpreventable tragedy by the father, blame often falls on the mother. Serious interactive difficulties may develop. Such problems may account in part, for the higher-than-normal incidence of divorce among SIDS parents. Consequently, where appropriate, the counselor should help the father understand and accept that there was nothing anyone could have done to prevent the death. In some instances, high credible sources, such as pediatricians, medical authorities, researchers, along with relevant literature (distributed by such organizations as the National SIDS Foundation) may facilitate the husband's acceptance of the fact that neither he nor his wife deserves blame. For example, in SIDS cases a teaching approach may be necessary, citing facts about babies who died of Sudded Infant Death in the arms of their fathers, mothers, doctors, even hospital personnel, and who, in every case, were diagnosed as victims of Sudden Infant Death Syndrome—meaning there was nothing anyone could have done to prevent the deaths. It is not uncommon for both fathers and mothers to have lingering doubts about the cause of death even after acceptance of the diagnosis of SIDS.

Verbalization of those doubts, in any childhood death event, does much to help clarify the problems caused by the death of the child. This verbalization is healthy for the self as well as imperative to the success of the relationship.

The traditional American family-role responsibility usually requires the husband to return to work immediately after the baby's death (of course, some mothers may also experience this temporal press). Many men express reluctance to return to normal work routine. It is in this environment that painful questions occur: "What did your baby die of?" "How did it happen?" Although the job structure may provide some distraction from grief, the male seldom has a retreat route at work; there is no place to grieve in private. To compound his problems, his co-workers often operate under the assumption that, after a few weeks, the grief process should be over and healing complete. For the parent, however, the painful memories and grief may linger on for years. To counteract these constrictions, the counselor must take steps to prepare working fathers for the inevitable questions. It can be explained that most people will know little about the cause of death, and their questions, although painful, are inquiries for understanding, not accusations. Although most people resolve memories of death due to disease relatively quickly, parents of children suffering from accidental death or SIDS often find the painful experience extends (or may recur) for many years. It should be emphasized, too, that this forgetting on the part of others does not indicate a lack of sensitivity or caring, but a need to return to normalcy.

There are some, albeit few, support services that counsel parents who have experienced the loss of a child by death. Within these organizations, however, it is rare to find male counselors. Organizations such as visiting, public, or community nurse associations, and the various parent contact groups frequently express the opinion that a male counselor or a male parent could interact more effectively than a female counselor. In fact, it is not uncommon for the male SIDS parent to walk out of the counseling session conducted by a female counselor. Whether this situation is a result of the man's attitude toward the counselor's gender, her occupation, or the topic of the death itself, is difficult to determine. Many counselors do report that when the male counselor is alone with the husband, interactive communication is generally achieved. The male-to-male identification may indeed be an important dimension to consider when scheduling a counseling session.

SUMMARY

For the male parent of a childhood death, it is imperative that the professional counselor provide the opportunity for catharsis by means of verbalization of his feelings about the death of his child. Fenichel (1945) stresses the need for the therapist to allow the patient to re-experience traumatic events, thus allowing for catharsis. Although it appears that female parents are more quickly able to retell the event and gain catharsis as a result, male parents have a much more difficult time. It is the father who exercises an unhealthy restraint of his emotions concerning the experience. And it is this same silent, strong male who fails to resolve his anger, pain, fears, and frustration over his loss. The counseling psychologist can facilitate the expression of these emotions and aid in developing a redefinition of self, which is a necessary prelude to the normal resolution of grief.

REFERENCES

Bergman, A.B. Sudden infant death syndrome. *Pediatric Clinics of North America,* 1974, *21*, 115–121.

Fenichel, O. *The psychoanalytic theory of neurosis.* New York: W.W. Norton, 1945.

Kübler-Ross, E. *On death and dying.* New York: Macmillan, 1969.

Woody, R.H. *Getting custody: Winning the last battle of the marital war.* New York: Macmillan, 1978.

The Male Spouse in Marital and Family Therapy

DAVID G. RICE

University of Wisconsin Medical School

The process of involving males in marital and family therapy and of facilitating their therapeutic growth presents special issues and problems. Some of these difficulties are similar to those faced by therapists in dealing with male clients in other forms of treatment, such as individual or group therapy. A major problem faced by the marital or family therapist is in getting the male spouse to actually come to therapy. One often gets the feeling that, in general, therapy is a more natural, and perhaps easier, experience for women than for men. Social conditioning has traditionally permitted women to show feelings openly and to reveal emotional pain directly to others. Indeed, more women than men seek psychotherapy (Chesler, 1972), and more commonly it is the wife who initiates marital or family therapy (Beck & Jones, 1973). In "traditional" marital relationships, this is a natural extension of assigning "expressive" functions to the wife and "instrumental" functions to the husband (Hicks & Platt, 1970). She is concerned with the emotional state of the family, he with the material state.

From a social-role-conditioning standpoint, the male spouse may feel as if he is entering marital or family therapy in a "one-down" position; not only is he likely to be "brought" rather than to have "sought" therapy but the arena and (verbal) weapons are more comfortable for his partner. In this sense, the reluctance of males to become readily involved in marital and family therapy is understandable. Yet, therapeutic outcome is likely to be more favorable if the spouses are seen conjointly (Gurman & Kniskern, 1978).

It has been the author's experience that a firm but reasonable insistence on having both partners present is usually effective in getting a reluctant spouse to come to the therapy sessions. This is achieved by explaining to the couple some of the possible risks of seeing only one partner—for example, differential spouse growth and change, lowered motivation to communicate and work on marital problems because one partner has an opportunity in therapy to talk these over, and the perception of a collusive alliance between one spouse and the therapist "against" the other spouse.

Once both partners are willing to enter therapy, there are other problems the marital or family therapist is likely to face. A case study will highlight some of these:

A couple requested therapy to help with an increasingly felt mutual dissatisfaction with their marital relationship. They had seen a woman therapist for approximately six months, but this ended when the husband took a job in another city. Both partners said that this experience "had not been very helpful," because the therapist had given "specific, direct advice" about problems they felt were "complex." Partly as a result of this experience, the couple had "shopped around" for another therapist and requested a "trial session" with the present therapist before making up their minds. The husband was 30 and the wife 28. They had two daughters, ages two and four months. He was employed in a professional civil service position and she had been an elementary school teacher, but stopped working just before the birth of their first child. He described his family background as "straight, upright, and somewhat cold, as far as affection goes." She described an "expressive, boisterous family, where everything was out in the open." Not surprisingly, the wife wanted more expressiveness on the husband's part, and he agreed this would be a good thing if he could do it. He indicated that he had no real complaints about her, although he felt ambivalent over the fact that she had stopped working and he was totally responsible for financial support of the family.

This couple was seen with a female co-therapist, who possessed an easy, genuine warmth, strong empathic abilities and a low-key, almost "folksy" manner. The therapists attempted from the start to create an atmosphere of minimal threat and refrained initially from challenging the couple's beliefs and defenses. However, both spouses displayed an unusual amount of resistance to the therapy process. There were many initial questions about fees, values, and beliefs (for example, "How do you feel about TA?," "How long will therapy last?," and "Is there any guarantee of success?"). The therapists, who despite the initial "hassles" felt an affinity toward both partners, tried to answer their questions patiently and honestly. Several attempts were made by the therapists to suggest that the degree of felt dissatisfaction with the marriage was probably equal for both spouses. The husband resisted this interpretation and seemed ready to accept that his inability to comfortably share feelings was "the problem."

The therapists noted that, in many ways, the husband put greater effort into, and received more "strokes" from his job than from his marriage. There he could exercise a fair amount of power in terms of directing and giving advice to other people. In this sense, his acceptance of himself as the "problem" and his capitulation to his wife's demand for "feelings": (a) served to reaffirm in her eyes that he "valued" a relationship (the marriage) that in actuality had come to play a less meaningful role in his life; and (b) protected him from having to express direct anger and felt frustration over her chronic expressions of dissatisfaction with him.

During the first six therapy sessions, the therapists attempted to get the husband to more directly and honestly express changes in his feelings toward his wife and how her "nagging" was alienating him. The male therapist shared some of his own frustration around the issue of balancing demands and rewards obtained from job and family. This was in part an attempt to help the husband realize that any felt alienation and irritation was not a totally unnatural response to his situation. The husband resisted the therapists' efforts and showed up alone for the seventh session. He said both partners had agreed that since the problem was "his" he should be coming to therapy. The woman therapist changed job assignments around this time and the male therapist continued to see the husband alone for sessions eight through ten. The male patient was able to express his feelings more directly with the male therapist than he had in the previous conjoint, co-therapy sessions. However, there was little indication that this behavior generalized to the marital relationship. The therapist suggested on several occasions that it would be more profitable if the wife came to some of the later sessions. Both resisted this idea and therapy ended when the husband did not show up for the scheduled eleventh session. Phone follow-up three months later indicated things were "OK" and that the couple was still together.

This case illustrates some common difficulties in involving male clients in the marital therapy process. Fortunately, the author has found most male clients in marital and family therapy are not quite so resistant to change. The modeling of feeling expression by both therapists and the permission to share ego-alien feelings within the therapy situation were only minimally effective in improving the marital relationship. Therapy seemed to help the husband become somewhat more comfortable with himself and to continue to do well in his job. However, in this couple the wife was defined as the "unhappy" one and the husband's motivation to change was more to "make her happy" than because he was dissatisfied with the way he was. His inability to express feelings as directly and openly as she would have liked was not a problem in his occupation. Thus, he had an "outside" source of ego gratification that enabled him to tolerate a certain degree of dissatisfaction within his marriage. He was accustomed in his job to a pattern of successful accomplishment with tangible results. Therapy, in contrast, with its emphasis on subjective "feelings" and subtle change, was frustrating and disillusioning for this man. At the point where he felt he had given it a reasonable chance (and, in that sense, had done what his wife had asked), he left therapy.

The above pattern of minimal therapeutic involvement, difficulty in handling feelings, having other powerful sources of reinforcement in one's life, and an inability to genuinely acknowledge responsibility for one's contribution to marital difficulties is a familar one. In dealing with these obstacles, which too often characterize male clients' behavior in marital and family therapy, the author has found certain techniques helpful. These include: (a) modeling the comfortable and direct expression of feelings, (b) defusing power and dominance issues, and (c) working with a co-therapist.

MODELING THE COMFORTABLE AND DIRECT EXPRESSION OF FEELINGS

The modeling of feeling expression, particularly by a male therapist, can be a powerful means for changing male clients' behavior. This takes advantage of the gender identification between therapist and client. However, the therapist must often make a special effort to promote this identification. If the wife sought out the male therapist "first," and then a conjoint family or marital session was arranged, an early identification with and transference of the wife to the male therapist may have been engendered. Even when the spouses are seen together from the start of therapy, the male therapist may establish a strong early positive countertransference relationship to the wife. She may relate somewhat more comfortably in therapy—for example, by opening up and talking more readily about feelings and problems. This can foster an affinity between the male therapist and the wife. This phenomenon occurs to a perhaps even greater degree for couples seeing a woman therapist. As a result of this process, the husband may perceive early in therapy a "collusion" between the therapist and his spouse to which he reacts defensively. He may become more withdrawn and silent, perhaps "pouting." Or he may put pressure on his spouse to leave therapy prematurely, saying in effect, "I don't believe therapy is going to help us any."

The therapist must be especially alert to this early "splitting" of husband and wife, based on the therapist's positive relating to the wife. Some of the "silence" shown by male clients in marital and family therapy may thus be induced by the therapist. Having male and female co-therapists can sometimes avoid these early collusive and splitting maneuvers, which leave one family member feeling alienated and without a perceived "ally" in therapy. However, the careful balancing of attention and effort toward each family member during the early part of therapy helps the therapist avoid this pitfall.

Once a positive therapeutic relationship is established with the male spouse, the male therapist's behavior can serve as a powerful model. If the therapist can express his own feelings directly and nondefensively, the male client can begin to see that such means of communication are "open" to men as well as to women. This can begin to undo some of the traditional masculine social/sexual role conditioning, which too often leads men to suppress and inhibit their emotional feelings. In addition, the therapist's capacity to tolerate productive silence in the therapy sessions and his or her ability to actively intervene through setting limits when needed and to subsequently "let go" of control when necessary for client growth are useful skills that the therapist can model.

There are many issues and problems that the therapist is likely to have struggled with in his or her own life that have the potential for profitable sharing with the male spouse in marital and family therapy. Primary among these would be incidents that illustrate the therapist's attempt to free himself or herself from the rigid constraints of traditional sex-role behaviors. For male therapists, in particular, it seems important to share something of their own initial apprehension over the resistance to the task of changing sex-role-prescribed behaviors, as well as some of the ultimate rewards of being able to change. It is helpful to point out that the therapist does not expect the client to become exactly like the therapist, but only to realize that they have shared in a common human struggle. It is also useful to point out that a person does not generally give up perceived social role power until he or she is convinced that there are advantages and rewards for doing so. Sharing the positive outcomes of this change process through the use of examples from the therapist's own relationships can promote client motivation for change. An example will help to illustrate this process:

> In many marriages the management of the family finances (budgeting, paying bills, and so forth) resembles a drawn-out ping-pong match. Responsibilities for this task are traded back and forth between husband and wife along the lines of "If you think you can do a better job, then here, it's all yours" or "He (or she) used to do that and it was a disaster" or "We each pay part of the bills and we seem, at times, to be working against one another." Recriminations fly back and forth, with the one whose current responsibility does not include managing the finances free to complain about what a "lousy job" the spouse is doing. The therapist's sharing of the way this is handled in his or her family can be useful, particularly if it is along the lines of: 'Well, in my family, one of us is not only willing to do that, but is probably better at it, so we let (me, her) do it. However, it took us a while to get there and we had some of the same struggles that you're having before we made the decision on the basis of preference and relative competence, rather than who needed to control or keep a rein on the other."

Admittedly, the therapist could have used "other families" (clients, friends, and so forth) to illustrate the above point, but the therapist's sharing of his or her own struggle and process of problem resolution may be more poignant and effective. The goal is to model for the male client flexible role behavior and sharing of power in the marital relationship without concomitant loss of self-esteem.

For many men, talking about feelings requires a certain letting go of power and control, with the risk of feeling weak and vulnerable. A helpful therapeutic strategy for "opening up" the affective area is to point out that most feelings are likely to be shown indirectly if they can't be expressed directly. Examples of the male client's passive-aggressive behaviors or his indirect communication of expectations—for example, in the sexual area—can help to concretize and validate this interpretation. In contrast to that which many men have been conditioned to expect, most wives are not "turned off" when their husbands show feelings. Indeed, these behaviors may be among the ones women are most likely to reinforce positively (Wills, Weiss, & Patterson, 1974); however, if such feeling expression on the husband's part is frightening or aversive to the wife, this must be dealt with first in therapy, before attempting to increase the level of affective communication between the partners.

The sharing of personal incidents where the therapist initially felt weak and vulnerable but subsequently gained some mastery of the situation can sometimes be helpful. An example will illustrate this:

> A couple in their early 30s entered marital therapy with complaints of increasing felt distance from one another over the last two of their seven years of marriage. They had a three-year old daughter. The husband had completed his professional training and taken a job with a high-pressure firm. He was doing well (partly at the expense of his marital relationship) but began to experience occasional chest pains. Only after a good deal of prodding from his wife was he able to talk about his fear of having a heart attack and dying. (A family history of coronary difficulties fed and compounded his fears.) After a thorough physical check-up, the symptoms were diagnosed as being most likely related to "anxiety." In the subsequent therapy session, both spouses began to talk about what they would do if one partner dies. The subject evoked considerable anxiety for both. They mentioned that neither had experienced the death of someone close to them. At this point, the therapist commented: "I think that's an important point. I used to feel quite frightened of the whole issue of death, until the unexpected death of my father, whom I was close to, was thrust upon me quite suddenly. It was, among other things, a shocking and scary reminder of my own mortality. But having to deal with his death, and working it through psychologically, has helped me to feel a little more confident about my ability to handle some previously very anxious feelings. (To husband) I think your recent episode with the chest pains may do something similar and I think it is important for both of you to continue talking about how you have been feeling about this."

HANDLING POWER AND DOMINANCE ISSUES

Previously the issue of the husband's possible felt powerlessness in the marital therapy setting was raised. Upon perceiving therapy to be the wife's "arena," the husband may attempt to restore his own sense of power either directly through dominating the sessions or indirectly through a variety of passive-aggressive resistance type behaviors—for example, by challenging the therapist repeatedly on minor interpretations and/or details about therapy procedures. In dealing with these power maneuvers, the therapist's ready willingness to share power within the therapy situation is important. A firm but nonauthoritarian posture on the therapist's part may be necessary.

The author has found it helpful with a verbally challenging and/or dominating male client to say something along the following lines: ''I have a feeling that we're in some sort of power struggle here and I sense both of us are feeling uncomfortable about it. You know, it's really no contest in the sense that you (the client) can very easily win. All you have to do is not talk or quit coming to therapy. But I don't think that would get either of us where we want to go.'' This statement re-emphasizes that the therapist and client must work together if therapy is to be successful. It further signifies that the therapist is willing to share power and is not threatened by the client's reasonable attempts to achieve a comfortable degree of control within the therapy situation. Working through this issue in therapy can have a good deal of carry-over for resolving power struggles in the marriage.

A willingness to share power in the marital relationship can be seen when the spouses are able to: (a) achieve a workable schedule for equitably dividing up domestic and child care responsibilities, (b) maintain important relationships with other people while not diminishing felt marital intimacy, and (c) allocate financial resources and responsibilities in a manner free of coercion and undue control by one spouse over the other. These tasks are elaborated and their facilitation through marital therapy discussed elsewhere (Rice & Rice, 1977).

WORKING WITH A CO-THERAPIST

The use of a co-therapist is often helpful in achieving many of the marital and family therapy goals with male clients alluded to in the previous sections. Male and female co-therapists can model a flexible pattern of relating, with open and direct communication of feelings and a comfortable sharing of power and control within the therapy situation. It is necessary for the co-therapists to have achieved a relationship that mirrors to some extent that seen as desirable for and by the clients. Otherwise, the couple's difficulties in communicating and relating may be magnified by the co-therapists' behavior rather than changed for the better. Each spouse has a potential ''ally'' in co-therapy, although these alignments tend to shift during therapy, depending on the issue. Thus, the problem of the male spouse feeling ''one-down'' in therapy can sometimes be avoided by the use of co-therapists and his motivation for participating and continuing in marital and family therapy thereby enhanced.

In summary, problems in involving the male spouse in marital and family therapy have been explored. Several techniques have been proposed for meeting these difficulties—namely, therapist modeling of the direct expression of feelings, use of a co-therapist, methods of defusing power and dominance issues, and therapist sharing of his or her own marital and family experiences. The emphasis has been on helping male clients toward greater flexibility of marital role behaviors and a more comfortable sharing of power within the family.

REFERENCES

Beck, D. F., & Jones, M. A. *Progress on family problems.* New York: Family Service Association of America, 1973.

Chesler, P. *Women and madness.* Garden City, New York: Doubleday, 1972.

Gurman, A. S., & Kniskern, D. P., Research on marital and family therapy; Progress, perspective, and prospect. In S. L. Garfield & A. E. Bergin (Eds.), *Handbook of psychotherapy and behavior change: An empirical analysis* (2nd ed.). New York: Wiley, 1978.

Hicks, M. W., & Platt, M. Marital happiness and stability: A review of research in the sixties. *Journal of Marriage and the Family,* 1970, *32,* 553–574.

Rice, D. G., & Rice, J. K. Nonsexist "marital" therapy. *Journal of Marriage and Family Counseling.* 1977, *3,* 3–10.

Wills, T. A., Weiss, R. L., & Patterson, G. R. A behavioral analysis of the determinants of marital satisfaction. *Journal of Consulting and Clinical Psychology,* 1974, *42,* 802–811.

INDEX